WHY CAN'T MY CHILD
STOP
EATING?

WHY CAN'T MY CHILD

STOP

EATING?

A GUIDE TO HELPING YOUR CHILD
OVERCOME EMOTIONAL OVEREATING

DEBBIE DANOWSKI

CENTRAL RECOVERY PRESS

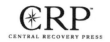

CENTRAL RECOVERY PRESS

Central Recovery Press (CRP) is committed to publishing exceptional materials addressing addiction treatment, recovery, and behavioral healthcare topics, including original and quality books, audio/visual communications, and web-based new media. Through a diverse selection of titles, we seek to contribute a broad range of unique resources for professionals, recovering individuals and their families, and the general public.

For more information, visit www.centralrecoverypress.com.
Central Recovery Press, Las Vegas, NV 89129

Publisher: Central Recovery Press
             3321 N. Buffalo Drive
             Las Vegas, NV 89129

Central Recovery Press makes no representations or warranties in relation to the medical information in this book; this book is not an alternative to medical advice from your doctor or other professional healthcare provider.

Characters portrayed in this book are composites, and all names thereof are fictitious.

18 17 16 15 14 13   1 2 3 4 5

ISBN: 978-1-937612-27-6 (paper)
      978-1-937612-28-3 (e-book)

Publisher's Note: Central Recovery Press books represent the experiences and opinions of their authors only. Every effort has been made to ensure that events, institutions, and statistics presented in our books as facts are accurate and up-to-date. To protect their privacy, the names of some of the people and institutions in this book have been changed.

Author's Note: A portion of the proceeds from this book will be donated by the author to H.O.R.S.E. of Connecticut, a nonprofit horse rescue organization located in Washington, CT. For more information about the organization, visit the website www.horseofct.org.

Cover design and interior layout by Heather Kern, Popshop Studio Design
Author photo by Patty Wahlers

Excerpts from *The Plug in Drug* by Marie Winn © 2002, Penguin Books. Used with permission.
Excerpt from *Addictive Thinking: Understanding Self-Deception* 2nd Edition by Abraham J. Twerski. Used with permission.

DEDICATION

This book is dedicated to overweight children everywhere.
May you all find health and happiness in your lives.

To all those who help abused and neglected animals.

TABLE OF CONTENTS

⬿

FOREWORD

❦

A PROFESSIONAL VIEW

THE TOPIC OF CHILDREN AND EATING IS important and timely. We live in an age in which childhood obesity rates are soaring while portion sizes in restaurants and fast-food outlets continue to grow, in which more children lead sedentary lives while the media promotes images of "perfect" bodies and faces, in which we receive confusing and often conflicting information about which diet (low-carb, high-fat? high-carb, low-fat? And what about protein?) is "best." It is hard for parents, let alone children, to even begin to make sense of the confusing and often contradictory messages we get in our society about food.

Eating behavior is the result of a complex interaction of genetics, sociological, and psychological factors. Research is just beginning to tease these apart. But what we do know—and what Dr. Danowski emphasizes in this book—is that eating behavior starts in the family, and that families play a powerful role in shaping children's eating habits. She understands the emotional stressors that both kids and parents experience in this complex world that often lead to overeating. For many, eating is a way of coping with life, even to the point where they are not able to know the difference between eating for biological reasons or eating for emotional solace.

As a clinical psychologist, psychology professor, and parent, one of my research specialties is emotional intelligence, which has to do, in part, with how people manage their feelings. In particular, I specialize in how children learn to handle distressing thoughts and feelings. I have run workshops and lectured to both parents and professionals on the development of emotional intelligence in children, helping children manage emotions, and emotionally intelligent parenting. Through my work as a clinical psychologist, I have come to believe that one of the most important things parents can teach their children is how to manage their emotions effectively. Within the psychological community, research has proven that one of the reasons some children overeat or develop eating disorders is because that is the only way they know to handle their emotions. Dr. Danowski's book provides readers with solid, concrete methods to address these emotional-eating issues.

As someone who has fought her own battle with food and who, through hard work, courage, and determination, has learned to change her relationship to food, Dr. Danowski is in a good position to understand the feelings of helplessness, loss of self-respect, and depression that people who struggle with food so often feel. In this book, she draws upon her own experiences as well as on research by others to discuss common reasons for overeating and what parents can do to help their kids.

She points out that healthy eating in children starts with parents and their own relationship to food. Although this is a book about children's eating habits, it is a book that speaks eloquently to parents and encourages them to examine their (often unconscious) beliefs about food and its role in their own lives. In fact, parents reading this book will find that they learn as much about themselves as about their children. As with so much in parenting, the reality is that parents can't be effective teachers and role models for their kids until they have examined the same issues in themselves.

In addition to providing sensible suggestions for changing patterns around food (including advice on food shopping, preparation, and presentation), Dr. Danowski discusses the psychological issues that often underlie eating. She points out what research has demonstrated, which is that disordered eating often stems from trouble with emotion management. Many people who eat excessively or who have eating disorders like anorexia and bulimia do not know how to identify or handle their feelings, particularly negative ones. They wind up turning to food to soothe and nurture themselves, sometimes at great expense to their physical health. Dr. Danowski provides important suggestions for helping kids identify and express the feelings that often lead to overeating.

This book provides an important way for parents to change their own and their children's relationship to food. The message is that food should be a way of nourishing the body, rather than a way of masking feelings or soothing oneself emotionally. As Dr. Danowski emphasizes, there are other positive ways to take care of one's emotional self. Parents reading this book will find not only that they are better educated about the role of food in children's lives but that they are in a better position to help children develop a healthy relationship to food.

Amy Van Buren, PhD

Clinical Psychologist

Associate Professor of Psychology

Sacred Heart University, Fairfield, CT

ACKNOWLEDGMENTS

WRITING A BOOK IS A TEAM EFFORT and this one is no exception. While it's impossible to acknowledge everyone who contributed to the making of this book, I'd like to mention several people who were especially instrumental in its publication. These include: my agent, Linda Konner, whose belief in my work has blessed my life immeasurably; my editor Helen O'Reilly, whose suggestions have made this a better book; the people at Central Recovery Press who worked hard to make this a reality; my writers group, who helped shape the initial proposal, Jessica Bram, Joanne Kabak, Jane Pollak and Lucy Hedrick; my colleagues at SHU and most especially those in my department, Jim Castonguay, Greg Golda, Lori Bindig, Sally Ross, Sid Gottlieb, Andrew Miller, and Suzanne Golub, who held things together for me during many challenging times.

My sister Karen and my niece Melissa; we have been through some difficult times together and are stronger and closer for it. My brother Mike and his wife Denise who have always been there when I needed them. My parents, who are no longer here. I hope you have found peace and happiness. My friends, Kelley Babbin, Matt Klebe, Susanna Madden, Beverly Robillard, Adria Perlman, Alex Minutillo, Ann Sieckhaus, Cinde and Wayne Soldan, who keep my head on straight when things get tough.

My farm friends—you have given my life a deeper meaning. Led by H.O.R.S.E. of Connecticut president Patty Wahlers, you have all changed my life: Mary Nelson, Ann Lynch, Anita Rusnak, Suzie Cosban, Dawn Hill, Ashley Nelson, Emily Slosson, John Livezey, Grace, Erin, John, Sena, Keith, Laura, Liz, Bob, Chris, Margot, Mary-beth, Olivia, Maddy, Val, Mike, John, and everyone one else who helps the horses. For Caramel who touched my heart in a special way, and all of the horses who have passed through the gates during my time there. Here's hoping for another 650 lives saved.

To my own animals who have brought so much joy into my life. Tiger Lily, my first pet, who knows when I need her. Tux, my beautiful boy, who is a survivor. Cooper, the one I couldn't let go home with anyone else but me, and sweet Butterscotch, who has taught me to be a better person.

And finally, to God, for the amazing life He has given me. I am so very grateful.

INTRODUCTION

❧

THEY NEVER LET HER DO ANYTHING FUN. Even though she was almost ten years old, Fiona's parents didn't allow her any freedom. Most of her friends were able to at least walk around the block in groups. Fiona's parents, however, refused to discuss the possibility until she was a teenager. It had been like this her whole life. Fiona's father had been a wild teenager, even serving jail time in his late teens. And though he had never been in trouble since, Fiona's father made sure that his daughter had little opportunity to repeat his mistakes.

"Fiona, it's time for dinner. Hurry up!" She could hear her mother's voice even though the music on her iPod was loud. Turning toward the window, Fiona could see her friends laughing and walking across the street. If it weren't for her stupid parents, then she would be there, too. Her friends were probably talking about what a baby she was, for not being allowed to take a simple walk around the block.

Grabbing her math book, Fiona flung it as hard as she could against the wall. Within seconds, Fiona's mother was at the door, banging.

"Fiona! Fiona! Are you all right? What was that crash?" As usual, her mother opened the door without waiting to be invited in.

"Nothing," Fiona glared at her mother.

She watched as her mother's eyes scanned the room. Fortunately, the book hadn't left a mark where it had hit the wall.

"Oh, well, okay. Come on then. Your dinner is getting cold. I made your favorite fried chicken and french fries." Fiona's mother smiled broadly then gently guided her in the direction of the kitchen.

Fiona knew that no one would yell at her for eating too much tonight; her parents always felt guilty whenever they refused to let her do something she wanted, and letting her eat whatever she wanted without comment was their way of making it up to her. Fiona was even planning on asking for a second helping of dessert. After that, she would sneak out of her bedroom while her parents were watching television and grab two snack-size bags of potato chips, being careful to fluff up the remaining packaging so as not to draw attention to the missing ones. Maybe her parents could stop her from seeing her friends, but Fiona wasn't going to let them stand between her and her food.

* * * * * * * *

AT TEN, FIONA HAS ALREADY DEVELOPED what will grow into a lifelong habit of associating happiness with unhealthy food. And a marketing savvy industry has created a customer for life among the ever-growing number of obese American children.

According to the U.S. Department of Health and Human Services, in the National Health and Nutrition Examination Survey, "the number of adolescents who are overweight has doubled since 1980 and the prevalence [of overweight/obesity] among younger children has more than tripled." Making matters worse is the amount of time these children will be obese. According to Dr. Roger Unger, an internist and professor at the University of Texas Southwestern Medical Center at Dallas, "Youngsters today will have been obese much longer than any preceding generation. The consequences could be deadly. Everybody talks about an epidemic, but they don't think about what it's going to be like twenty years from now when these kids are approaching middle age and have heart disease and all sorts of complications of diabetes."

Despite all of the current efforts, obesity rates in children are climbing with no end in sight. Is it because parents don't care enough about their children? Of course not. Something is missing in their efforts. But what is it? Certainly it's not a lack of nutritional information. Newspapers, magazines, and television programs are filled with information about healthy eating. Bookstore shelves and pediatricians' offices overflow with advice about properly feeding children. Yet, nothing seems to help. Why?

While most of us know what constitutes a healthy meal, very few are aware of the emotions behind the food that is presented to children on a regular basis. And even fewer understand how these emotions are entangled with childhood overeating.

Think about how foreign it would seem for you to celebrate your birthday without a cake. How about getting through a holiday without baking and/or eating special desserts? Think about your childhood. Did one or both of your parents or grandparents have a special food that they made for you, or was there a certain treat that you were permitted only when you were ill or unhappy, one that was supposed to make you feel better?

Even though all of these things may seem like normal childhood behaviors and none of them is necessarily harmful in moderation, there are emotions attached to each event. For instance, having a cake made specifically for your birthday makes you feel special and loved. Eating dessert is often associated with family love (for some) or as a shield against explosive family gatherings for others. And being given special food as a child may be related to feelings of love and nurturing. This being so, is it any wonder that obesity is becoming a "national scandal," as one expert notes?

It is the intention of *Why Can't My Child Stop Eating?* to first create awareness about the current attitudes and practices in society that contribute to emotional overeating in children; then, to provide concrete actions to initiate and maintain lifestyle changes. Since this issue is so crucial to the health and development of children, helping parents help their children heal from the emotional aspects of obesity by addressing these issues and providing practical activities is vitally important.

This book is also designed with busy parents in mind. It is intentionally kept short so that you will have time to read all of it. Chapters 2–6 contain a "Things to Remember" section that summarizes the main points of each chapter. This is to reinforce what you have already read. It is not designed to replace reading the entire chapter. There are many things in each chapter that are not included in the "Things to Remember" sections. Think of these sections as a quick reference guide for after you have read the entire chapter.

And though many may point to genetics as the cause of childhood obesity, it is important to remember that according to a nursing professor at Michigan State University, the majority of overweight cases— approximately 60 to 80 percent—are due to lifestyle, while only 20 to 40 percent have genetic causes. This being so, the rate of childhood obesity can be greatly reduced with the lifestyle changes outlined in *Why Can't My Child Stop Eating?*

CHAPTER ONE

⁓

SOCIETY, FOOD, AND EMOTIONAL EATING

TAKING A DEEP BREATH, I DUG MY fingers into the palms of my hand. I knew what was coming. Within a matter of a few seconds I would be assaulted. Forcing myself not to look in the direction of the teenagers gathered in front of the garage on the corner, I said a silent prayer that they wouldn't notice me, especially today in front of Linda, a girl in my grade for whom my mother occasionally babysat and who walked home with me after school on the days she came to our house.

My heart began to pound as I bit my lower lip to stop the tears that were welling up in my eyes. I forced myself to try and concentrate on what Linda was saying. Though I saw her mouth moving, I had no idea what the words were. Then I heard the high-pitched voices call out.

"Look at the whale! Why doesn't she go back to the ocean?" Laughter filled the air.

"Fat ass. Lose weight." Again, the laughter.

Walking as fast as my layers of fat would allow, I kept my head high and focused my eyes straight ahead, digging my front teeth even harder into my lower lip. I knew my eyes would betray me, so I avoided

Linda's gaze and prayed that she wouldn't tell anyone else about this. It wasn't as if she was a friend. I barely knew her. Like everyone else at school, she stayed away from me.

"That's so disgusting. How could anyone let themselves get so fat?" I heard the deep voice behind me.

My knees shook as I prayed that my legs wouldn't give out underneath me. If I fell now, in front of "them," I would surely die of embarrassment. A few more steps and I could no longer hear the laughter I knew was still there.

Reaching my house, I pulled at the front door handle, rushing in before Linda. Unclenching my fists and letting my shoulders droop, I exhaled slowly. I was home. I was safe.

Clearing my throat, I looked at my mother.

"Maybe you can make us Mommy Burgers so Linda can try one." I used my sweetest voice. My mother hesitated only for a second before her eyes filled with sympathy, and then she nodded her head.

I could feel the saliva gathering in the corner of my mouth as I thought about the two cheeseburger patties sandwiched between three slices of white bread, slathered with gobs of mayonnaise on one side and ketchup on the other. I knew that since we had company, my mother would do as I requested—even allowing me to eat two.

As I bit into the thick sandwich, my whole body relaxed. Even if no one else in the world liked me, I knew that my mother loved me. No matter what I did or how fat I was, she would always be there. Smiling at my mother, I hoped she would give us dessert next . . . .

To my parents, and so many other members of their generation, a fat child was a healthy child. Coming from times and places that had experienced deprivation and want such as a Great Depression survived by my grandparents and the aftermath of World War II when my parents lived through food rationing, they embraced a cultural ethos that told them that the preparation and presentation of food was not only necessary for survival, it was a demonstration of love. And so they fed me accordingly.

As a child, I believed that the more food my parents bought and prepared for me the more they loved me. As I grew older and moved from the haven of family to the bigger world of the classroom, eating became a way of coping with the pain I experienced as the fattest child in elementary school. And though I didn't know it at the time, I was setting myself up for a lifetime of emotional eating that would eventually result in my reaching a top weight of 328 pounds. Growing up in a time when treatment for eating disorders and individual counseling were looked at as stigmatizing a family's reputation, I never imagined that there was any other way to deal with my emotions.

On television, I saw mothers who regularly baked cookies to show love for their children. I studied the way these families gathered at the dinner table to discuss the events of the day, all while enjoying a mouthwatering meal lovingly prepared by Mom. And during the commercial breaks, I saw toys intertwined with food, too—my favorite being a real, working oven whose heat supply was a light bulb. With this little jewel, I could actually bake and frost a real cake. Then, there were the cereal boxes, each containing a prize. I could barely contain myself, finishing the sugary flakes in record time to reach the plastic treasure.

In books, I read about Nancy Drew and the delectable meals she and her father shared, oftentimes inviting her boyfriend Ned and best friends George and Bess. To me, this was the ultimate in true friendship—being able to eat in front of friends without worrying about what they would think.

In real life, I knew that if I went to the dentist, the doctor, or even the bank, the receptionists or tellers there would have candy or a lollipop for me if the experience was stressful or there was a long wait. They all did their best to make my visit more pleasant. This was great—but holidays were the best. For weeks before these special days, my mother and grandmothers would bake cookies and cakes that I only got to eat once or twice a year. Christmas was my favorite because there was even more food around than during any of the other holidays, and my grandmother baked a particular Italian delicacy—something she only did once a year.

* * * * * * * *

DID I HIDE THE PAIN AND SHAME of the teasing I endured because I didn't trust my parents? No. In fact, it was nearly the opposite—I didn't want to worry them. I grew up knowing that my parents were desperately concerned about the size of my body. They always did whatever they could to try to encourage me to lose weight. I truly believe that either one of them would have given a limb if it would have solved my problem.

I approach this book with the knowledge that whether or not you are a parent of an overweight child, a stepparent, a grandparent, a guardian, an aunt or uncle, or a close friend, you share the same concern for the child in your life that my parents had for me. You are probably willing to do whatever you have to in order to help your child become healthier, yet it is my guess that you have been bombarded with so much information that you are uncertain about how to proceed. I know this because as a twenty-three-year-old adult, I was faced with the same situation. I had tried just about every diet program out there and had failed. I didn't know what was missing in my efforts and was completely overwhelmed by the amount of weight-loss information available.

Through intensive individual and group counseling and even by spending six weeks of my life in inpatient psychiatric treatment, I eventually discovered that I had, and have, a physical addiction to sugar, flour, and caffeine—a concept that was quite unknown during the late 1980s. With a lot of hard work, I was able to turn my life around but at a very severe cost. Choosing good health for myself today, one day at a time, means accepting I cannot eat items that contain large amounts of sugar, flour, or caffeine.

To maintain my recovery, I weigh and measure my food and plan each and every bite that goes into my mouth. Though extreme, this is the only thing that has ever worked in my life. For the past twenty-three years, I have enjoyed a 150-pound weight loss and lived a relatively normal life which is not adversely affected by food and eating. I choose to live this way, one day at a time, in order to maintain my hard-won health.

What does all of this have to do with you, the child in your life, and this book? For starters, this book is an attempt to save your child from experiencing the intense pain of recovery from a full-fledged addiction. As a child, I was unaware of the ways that I used food to deal with my emotions. For me, food was comfort. It was my friend, my lover, and even my confidante. No matter what was happening in my life, I felt that I would get through it—as long as I had my food. Overeating was as natural to me as breathing.

At the time, I didn't realize that I was planting the seeds of addiction by using food to deal with my emotions. The concept of emotional eating, though gaining more popularity today, was never even a consideration when I was a child. My parents simply did what they had learned from their parents, who did what they had learned from their parents, and so on. No one had the knowledge to realize that emotional eating could be dangerous to children and to society as a whole.

Today, though the concept of emotional eating is gaining more attention—as evidenced by appearances like the one I made on the FOX Cable News show *The O'Reilly Factor*, during which I discussed the topic—there is little, if any, information about specifically helping your child to overcome his or her emotional eating. Similarly, although there are several well-written and respected books about the societal attitudes that contribute to overeating (*Food Politics: How the Food Industry Influences Nutrition and Health* by Marion Nestle, and *Food Fight: The Inside Story of the Food Industry, America's Obesity Crisis, and What We Can Do About It* by Kelly D. Brownell and Katherine Battle Horgen are two good examples), there is little information about changing emotional eating patterns in children. This book aims to change that.

In these pages, you will not find a recommended food plan for your son or daughter, nor will you find growth charts telling you what your child should weigh. Bookstore shelves and pediatricians' offices are filled with this information, so it can be easily obtained. Rather, this book will concentrate on addressing the emotional issues that are tied to eating and food. While most of us know what constitutes a healthy meal, how many of us are aware of the emotions behind the food that we present to children on a regular basis?

Societal solutions, though alluded to in these pages, are not the focus of this book. You, the reader, whether as an individual family member or friend of an overweight child, will find here specific suggestions that you can take to improve the quality of that child's life by severing the link between emotional connection and food.

Because this information may be new to you, and may at times seem radical or unusual, it's important that you prepare yourself before you read on. First, please know that the single most important thing you can do while reading this is to stop blaming yourself for your child's situation. It's vital that you are aware of this tendency right up front. As you will discover, there are many societal attitudes that contribute to emotional eating. You did not invent these, nor are you responsible for them. Once you've read the information in this book, you can make a decision about what you will change; but it is never okay to punish yourself for things you think you've done wrong. As a parent, you did the very best you could with what you knew. Once you know more, you can change your patterns.

Second—please keep an open mind. Some of the concepts you will read will be unfamiliar to you and may seem extreme. Try to remain open to the suggestions. Remember, you are questioning societal attitudes that have been pervasive for decades. These attitudes are ingrained in our culture—they have in some instances become part of the traditions and observances we celebrate and enjoy as Americans. This being said, keep in mind that serious problems require serious solutions. If you have truly tried everything you can think of to help your child with little success, then you owe it to yourself and your child to open your mind to the information presented here. It may be the only chance you have to save your child from the life I described above.

In tandem with this, though you may be tempted to put all of these suggestions into action immediately, that is not a good idea. Throughout this book, you will be reminded to choose one or two areas to work on rather than trying to do everything. Decide what you consider to be your child's most troublesome area and work on that. If you attempt to change everything all at once, you will create resentment in your child and perhaps even in yourself. This will not only be counterproductive, it will make your efforts seem haphazard and thus ineffective. The size of the effort is not nearly as important as the consistency behind it. One small and consistent change will mean more than ten sporadic ones. Keep in mind that big journeys begin with small steps.

As you continue to read, you will learn more about how to deal with the "saying-no-to-food" guilt. For right now, think about many of the ways that food is used as something other than a means of nourishing human bodies. It would be very helpful for you to make a list of those ways that may be present in your child's life that food is used for a purpose other than nutrition. Here are some ideas to get you started. (Remember, the items listed here are not the only ways food is used to deal with emotions.)

- A baby cries and a parent automatically reaches for a bottle.
- A child goes to the doctor for a shot and is presented with a lollipop afterward.
- A preschooler learns to bake cookies as a classroom activity.
- A child is threatened with "no dessert" if the entire plate of food is not eaten.
- A kindergartener is bribed with an ice cream cone for good behavior during a haircut.
- A filled cookie jar sits on the kitchen counter in one family's home to serve as a reward for good behavior to the children who live there.
- An elementary school child's parents are asked to provide cupcakes to celebrate their child's birthday in class.
- A yearly family activity involves making cookies for Grandma's birthday.
- Following a day of outdoor activities, school children are

presented with ice cream.

- Middle school students taking part in a musical play convene after the performance to eat cake and cookies at the wrap party.
- A child invites others over to a pizza birthday celebration.
- A high school student puts money in a vending machine to buy two candy bars for a quick lunch so she has more time to talk to the boy she likes.
- Stressed-out over constant bickering, a parent relents, giving a teenager $20 to have dinner out with friends.
- After a relationship breakup, a high school student eats a half-gallon of ice cream.
- Watching television cooking shows is a regular part of one family's routine.

Does any one of these sound familiar? If not, were you able to come up with your own list? Whatever you found, take a moment to look it over. Are you surprised? How many of the items on your list did you do as a child? What about your parents? Do you know if they, too, did those things as children?

Don't worry if you weren't able to make a long list or couldn't answer all of the previous questions. Later in the book, you will be asked to write more about this. Right now, the important thing is for you to begin thinking about the role food plays in your child's life.

While you are contemplating all of this, think, too, about the fact that as a society, we give lip service to the idea that fruits and vegetables are important for our health, whereas our actions indicate that we value the flavor of fatty, high-calorie foods more because of their taste. "Remember, actions speak louder than words."

While many parents would assert that they value fruits and

vegetables, think for a minute exactly how that value is demonstrated. In many families, a great deal of energy is expended urging children to eat healthy foods, including fruits and vegetables. Sometimes even threats or bribes are used to accomplish this. Yet, how frequently do parents in these families actually model the behavior—eating fruits and vegetables—themselves? Or, if a parent tells a child to eat all of his or her vegetables so that he or she can have dessert, then the subtle message being sent is that dessert is more desirable than the actual meal. Dessert becomes a reward to be eaten only after a chore (eating vegetables) is accomplished.

Similarly, when a child is rewarded with special foods after accomplishing a difficult task or attending to an unpleasant event, the unconscious message is that the "reward foods"—usually high-calorie dessert items—are a means of soothing unpleasant feelings. Or, if a child's school uses dessert items to celebrate birthdays and holidays, the lesson being imparted is that these items are more desirable than the everyday foods he or she regularly eats. This creates a food hierarchy wherein certain items are more important than others. Let's consider what can happen when children are given these messages.

A child who receives the message that high-calorie dessert items are a form of comfort during difficult times will continue to turn to these when life becomes unpleasant. In the same way, a child taught to use these items to celebrate special events will become dependent on certain foods to have fun or receive satisfaction from life. Taken to the extreme, this behavior could lead to obesity, even death.

Though many of these social practices were established years before the current rise in obesity, the difference now is due to the extent and the combinations involved. Unlike in years past, today's children are faced with a greater number of fears and challenges than ever before: rapid technological progress, the threat of war, unemployment, inflation, rising health care costs, extremely high beauty standards, child molestation, a rise in the number and degree of violent crimes, rising divorce rates, etc. The list could go on forever but the point is that children today are faced with numerous challenges. How many of us worried about even half of the things on this list when we were growing up? Quite the contrary to our experiences, children and young adults today regularly worry about most of the things mentioned.

For instance, graduating from high school no longer guarantees that teens will get good jobs or be successful. In fact, great pressure is put on today's students to begin preparing for college admission in elementary school, with the result that a grade of B can be a cause for tears if the child in the next seat gets an A. Most children are subjected to the pressures of standardized tests well before entering their junior year in high school, while some begin as early as middle school to plan their college majors.

Those who dream of getting married can no longer look forward to a "happily EVER after." Quite the opposite, as more than half of those marrying will end up in divorce courts within a few years. Children and adolescents are well aware of this.

Now, think for a second about children's schedules today (and it's only recently that such words as "children" and "schedule" would have been written in the same sentence). In the past, childhood was a time of freedom and of "making one's own fun." By contrast, today's children are shuffled from activity to activity (music lessons, scout meetings, team sports, religious education, private instruction in a variety of subjects, etc.) in an effort to make them well-rounded adults and give them an edge in applying to college. Little, if any, time is left over for children to simply entertain themselves. The leisure time left gets eaten up by television and computers, neither of which involve the kind of meaningful physical activity that contributes to a fit frame, while at the same time standards for physical beauty have never been higher, for both boys and girls.

Interestingly enough, the recent rise in—and fear of—obesity among children has promoted a "look good on the outside" mindset. Today, even infants are provided with designer clothing. Store shelves abound with children's makeup, nail polish, cologne, "sexy" underwear for young children, and so forth. The pressure for children to "look good" has never been greater.

Add to all of this the current state of the American family. Even children in two-parent families are aware of the negative effects of divorce. It is no longer guaranteed that both parents will be in a child's life on a daily basis. Yet, children's television programs and movies are filled with images of supposedly "perfect" two-parent families, much as they have been for generations. Thanks to endless reruns, today's children are exposed to the same unrealistically divorce-free, intact-family-celebrating programming that their grandparents viewed.

Take for example, the fact that on several cable stations you can regularly view the programs that were popular when the Baby Boomers were youngsters. These stations regularly air repeats of shows such as *The Brady Bunch* and *The Partridge Family*. Though neither family has traditional roots (the Bradys are a blended family, created after both partners were widowed, and the Partridges do not have a traditional father present) both have strong, nurturing male and female characters. In the case of the Bradys, both parents are regularly available for the children while the Partridges have a strong mother and a nurturing father figure (the family's band manager). Neither program makes allowances for the absent mothers or fathers who have become realities in today's children's lives. The fact that such television families are far from universal is never explained to the children who make up much of the television audience. No wonder that many children feel there is something wrong with their own families when viewed alongside such models of togetherness. That feeling of not being "normal" or even "good enough" can add to a child's stress.

A real-life example of using food to deal with the stress of divorce comes from Sean, a child who began to overeat after his parents divorced. After moving to a new house, starting a new school, and seeing his father only on weekends, Sean began to overeat and watch an excessive amount of television, resulting in the seven-year-old's ballooning to ninety-six pounds at four feet tall.

"I think maybe I contributed to the weight thing because I was so emotionally stressed about this divorce," says his mother, Val. "I wanted him to feel okay, so I didn't deny him anything." Because children began teasing him, Sean finally asked his mother to help him lose weight.

As if school and family stressors aren't enough, crimes against children are on the rise. It wasn't too long ago that new mothers simply left their babies sleeping in their car seats for a quick run into the store. Today, this notion sends shivers down the spines of parents everywhere—and rightly so. To leave a child unattended in public for any length of time greatly increases the odds that the child will be harmed or even kidnapped. (And to leave an unattended child in a car is to risk his or her death from overheating or at the very least, a fine or public censure for the parent.) Young children are regularly fingerprinted for identification in case of foul play, and milk cartons and mail inserts are filled with pictures of missing children. No matter how hard parents may try to shield them, children and young adults are aware of the dangers surrounding them.

Put all of these stressors together—high academic expectations, overbooked schedules, more rigorous beauty standards, rising divorce rates, and increased crime against children—and you have some idea of the issues facing today's children. In general, the emotional state of the country, and specifically of children, is chaotic and filled with fear. Now, more than ever, nurturing is needed to deal with the issues mentioned above. Unfortunately, many of today's children are learning to nurture themselves by overeating.

Think for a moment about the many ways in which children are taught to use food to make themselves feel better. How many times has your child been offered a lollipop, cookie, or ice cream after a doctor's visit, or a special comfort food like mashed potatoes or mac'n'cheese when he or she is sick?

Modern, Western parents no longer fear starvation, for themselves or their children. But it wasn't so long ago that food was scarce. It was not uncommon for people to suffer from and even die of malnutrition. Eating was therefore seen as a means of promoting health, and a fat child was seen as a healthy child. While our societal circumstances have changed, our attitudes have not. Food is still used to nurture children during difficult or stressful times. The biggest difference now, however, is that the abundance of foods high in fat and calories allows children to eat a greater variety and a more dangerous quantity of food to nurture themselves.

In addition to using food to soothe our children, we also use it to reward good behavior. The practice of using lollipops after a trip to the doctor or dentist, though fortunately being phased out in most modern medical and dental practices, continues in others. Even though this may seem innocuous enough, let's consider for a second the unconscious message being sent to children. When food is used as a reward, children are given the idea that eating is associated with the good feelings of being rewarded. By making food a reward, we teach children to place too great a value on eating. Rather than sending the message that eating is a biological act needed to nurture our bodies, children are regularly taught that food is a reward for good behavior, thus setting up a form of competition between those foods considered desirable and those that are healthy, or, even more dangerous—the expectation that all good behavior will be rewarded with treats.

Consider for a moment that a child with this expectation misbehaves in the grocery store. In the past, he or she has been bribed to discontinue such behavior with a sweet treat. If given a cookie or candy, this child has learned that food is provided for a desired behavior—he or she has also learned how to manipulate others in order to receive high-calorie foods, thus setting up a dangerous cycle as the child grows. Imagine this child as a teenager who has just completed a difficult homework assignment or gotten a good grade on a test. What do you think he or she will desire as a reward? Even more alarming, how many times in his or her life do you think food will be used in this manner?

Taking this a step further, one of the most dangerous ways that food is used is as a means of showing love. While this concept is related to the previous discussion of using food to nurture, there is an important distinction here. Using food to show love means that children come to associate, perhaps even confuse, parental or familial love with food. Therefore, when a child feels unloved, he or she may seek out food. Taken to an extreme, this may result in morbid obesity at a very young age.

Rather than learning to deal with feelings of rejection or lack of affection in healthy ways, when food is used as love, children become conditioned to reach for food. As time goes on, children will grow into adults unable to distinguish between eating for biological reasons and eating for emotional solace. It's important to read the previous sentence once again. The danger of using food to satisfy emotions lies in the fact that children (and later adults) become unable to recognize genuine feelings of hunger. Without knowing what physical hunger feels like, children are unable to use food in the manner for which it was intended—to nourish their bodies.

In addition to all of the feelings children often associate with food and eating in their families, there are many unhealthy messages presented through the media. On any given Saturday morning, children's cartoons are filled with commercials for fast and junk foods targeted to convince young minds into believing that fun can be had by consuming these products. One of the biggest examples of this is the creation of cultural icons designed to appeal to children. The biggest of the fast-food giants have their happy-go-lucky clown and their rambunctious king, and candymakers have even animated the candy-coated chocolate figures that "melt in your mouth, not in your hands," sending them to parties, and even having them go trick-or-treating in commercials. Many candy commercials depict ordinary children at play.

Though these kinds of advertisements have been around for years and have come to be accepted as part of society, most people have never thought about the messages being sent to children. When a group of children or young adults appears in commercials, eating chips or candy while laughing and having fun, viewers are given the subtle—and sometimes not so subtle—message that eating these high-calorie items will add fun and excitement to their lives. Yet the reality is actually quite different. Eating these items will cause children to gain weight, thus making them unable to participate in the portrayed activities.

Taking all of this information and putting it together, it is easy to see how children have come to associate food and eating with many emotions and actions. Using food to nurture children, as a reward, to show love, and to help them experience fun and freedom, puts greater importance on food than necessary. And when food is used to deal with or express feelings, children do not learn healthy coping skills. Rather, a child who knows only food as a means of coping with stress, expressing emotions, or nurturing is more likely to turn to eating to deal with life's problems.

Now, add to this the fact that inactivity, likely due to television and Internet use, is increasing and physical education classes are being cut or downsized and the problem becomes even more serious. According to the most recent study by the U.S. Department of Health and Human Services, available at the organization's website (http://aspe.hhs.gov), "Schools are decreasing the amount of free play or physical activity that children receive during school hours. Only about one-third of elementary children have daily physical education, and less than one-fifth have extracurricular physical activity programs at their schools. Daily enrollment in physical education classes among high school students decreased from 42 percent in 1991 to 25 percent in 1995, subsequently increasing slightly to 28 percent in 2003. Outside of school hours, only 39 percent of children ages 9–13 participate in an organized physical activity, although 77 percent engage in free-time physical activity."

Furthermore, according to statistics from the U.S. Department of Health and Human Services at the National Diabetes Information Clearinghouse, approximately 215,000 people younger than twenty years of age have diabetes. Among those twenty years or older, 1.9 million people were newly diagnosed with diabetes in 2010. Approximately

20,000 youths each year are diagnosed with diabetes. This number is expected to increase.

While many point to genetics as the reason for the problems discussed in this chapter, two researchers disagree and point out that society and the cultural environment contribute greatly. The associate director of the division of nutrition at Harvard Medical School points out that genetics in humans have only experienced small changes. As previously noted, 20 to 40 percent of overweight cases are attributable to genetics, and 60 to 80 percent to lifestyle. If we accept this as true, and I do, the rate of childhood obesity can greatly be reduced by making lifestyle changes.

Though the last sentence is the key to successfully helping your child to stop emotionally overeating, please remember that you don't have to make these lifestyle changes all at once. If you've read all of the information in this chapter, you've already "digested" a great deal. You may be feeling overwhelmed, or even worse, ineffective as a parent. Realize that these thoughts are quite normal but at the same time think about the fact that they may not be true. Whenever a person begins something new, his or her subconscious feels threatened. The way that the subconscious manages these threats is by using fear or negative thinking as a way to prevent further action.

In other words, since you first began reading this, your subconscious has been in protection mode, attempting to keep your current life intact. This is accomplished by trying to sabotage any new efforts you make at improving your life. Try to think of your subconscious as the voice of a scared child. When a child feels threatened, he or she is likely to "act out," saying and doing negative things to try and feel in control of the situation. It's the same with your subconscious. When the *status quo* of your life seems threatened with change, whether for the better or not, a part of your mind kicks into action to stop something—anything—new from happening.

You are at that point right now. Your mind is telling you all of the reasons why you shouldn't even begin to undertake changing your child's eating habits. And it is doing so in a very subtle way. The voices inside of your head probably aren't denying the fact that your child's eating habits need improvement. Instead, they are finding things to criticize about the information you've just read. They are telling you that this will be too much work or that you don't have the time. Or perhaps your inner voices are saying that your child isn't "that bad" or doesn't need help. Rather than listen to your voices, consider the following example.

At thirteen, Dana was nearly twenty-five pounds overweight and miserable. Unable to participate in many of the same activities that her normal-weight friends did, Dana often turned to food as way of handling the sadness she felt. Though her well-meaning mother regularly tried to limit her intake of junk food, the result was disastrous. Dana, feeling out of control in her life, was determined to have power over her eating no matter how destructive it was. Every time her mother prohibited her from eating high-calorie foods, Dana sneaked food without her mother's knowledge. The two were at odds with no hope of making any progress.

Desperate to get her daughter help, Dana's mother decided to follow several of the suggestions outlined in this book. First, she had an honest conversation with her daughter about the health risks of obesity. Then, she began to concentrate on being a good role model by eating healthier herself. And, finally, Dana's mother offered her daughter several options for changing her eating habits. Rather than impose strict guidelines, Dana's mother let her child have a say in solving her problem. Even more important, Dana's mother made sure that her daughter was provided with alternative ways of dealing with the emotions that she regularly ate over.

Today, Dana is a happy, well-adjusted teenager who is living life to the fullest. She no longer needs to overeat and has since learned to eat healthy meals. Dana also made exercise a regular part of her routine. Now, at a normal weight, Dana is enjoying a life she never could have imagined several months ago.

This was only possible because her parents took actions that were unfamiliar, even frightening, at times. Now, it's your turn. Are you ready to help change your child's life? If so, read on and find out how.

CHAPTER TWO

❦

IT BEGINS WITH YOU

THOUGH YOU HAVE CHOSEN THIS BOOK TO help your child, in this chapter you will be asked to answer some questions about and to examine your own eating behaviors. While you may be resistant, it's important to remember a few things before continuing. Despite the fact that you are presented with pointed questions, none of the information here or anywhere else in this book is designed to place blame on you or your parenting skills. It is a waste of energy to squander time thinking about blaming anyone for your child's situation. Quite the opposite, you are reading this book to help your child. That, alone, shows how much you care for the welfare of your child's future. A saying from the rooms of twelve-step recovery comes to mind: "If we knew better, we would do better." Let yourself off the hook for behaviors you may have engaged in before you "knew better."

This being said, it's vital that you recognize the patterns in your eating behaviors that have been passed on from your own parents and from their parents. The best way to think of this comes from a lecture given by a famed physician who said that we shouldn't blame our parents for the dysfunction that is present today. They only did what their parents taught them and their parents did what their parents taught them. The doctor says that we should blame Adam and Eve for starting it all!

Even though this is a humorous example designed to make a point, the idea presented is worth noting. Each set of parents did—and is doing—the best that they knew how and as time goes on, each generation becomes more aware of the harmful habits and makes an effort to change them. Now, it's your turn.

The only way to change something, however, is to first be aware of it. This is true of everything, from recovery from addiction to unhealthy eating habits. This is where your own eating habits come in. If you don't identify the patterns in your family, then you can't make the necessary changes in your attitudes and behaviors to help your child. In other words, if you don't know what you're doing, then you can't change it.

Before continuing, it's also important to remember that you will not be able to change everything all at once—nor should you try. The point here is to become aware of your actions and the dynamics of the family situation, not to immediately run out and change everything. Some things will remain the same no matter how hard you try. That's okay. Others will be easier to change or alter and these are the ones on which you should first concentrate your attention. If you start to feel overwhelmed by the questions here, take a short break to give yourself time to process what you are learning. But be sure to come back, as what you are discovering is vital to the health of your child.

To begin, take a few minutes to think about your own childhood. What role did food play in your life? You may want to take out a pen and paper to make some quick notes so that you don't forget (a special notebook to use while reading this book might be helpful). While writing, think about how your parents used food. Did your mother always cook a special meal for your birthdays? Was your father there to take you out for ice cream every week? If so, what feelings did you associate with these events? Did you consider these or other activities as a way of feeling loved? Were you treated in a special way during these times? Take a moment to complete the following sentence, "In my family, food was a way of . . . ."

Now, take a moment to think of the feelings about food you had as a child. Don't go back and read anything you've written so far. Just keep right on writing. There will be time for reading later. Right now, you need to simply write as much as you can. When you were younger, how did you feel about food? Was it a way of relaxing? Feeling special? Getting rewarded? Nurturing yourself when things didn't go your way? Celebrating? Whatever you thought about food then, write it down and don't worry about making it "pretty." There's no need for spelling or grammar review at this point. Simply write as much as you can, in any way that you can. If you're better with a computer or you'd like a certain type of pen, then by all means do whatever feels comfortable to you while you are writing.

After you have finished the exercise above, write about one incident in your childhood involving food that stands out in your memory. Was this incident a happy one? Were you sad? Did you feel loved? Whatever it was, simply write it down without rereading it. By now you will probably need a break. Feel free to get up and walk around, or maybe even wait until tomorrow morning to come back to your writing. While you are doing other things, be aware of the thoughts that come up. During your break time, your subconscious will be thinking about what you've written. By the time you come back to your writing, you will most likely have new things to add.

Before proceeding, take some time to write down any memories involving food (or lack of food) that may have come into your mind. Don't worry if you're unsure of what they mean right now. The important thing is to write as much as you can about your childhood and the role food played in your family while you were growing up.

Though your first reaction may be to minimize certain events that come up, simply write them down for now. If it came up in your mind during this exercise, then chances are that there is something there you can use.

Rather than viewing this as an indictment of your childhood and/or your parents, try to think of yourself as a detective attempting to solve a mystery. Your past is simply that, your past. It can't be changed, and the information you find doesn't have to change the life you have today unless you decide it is necessary. For the moment, it may help to look at your life as if it were a movie or television show. Other than naming the feelings involved with the experiences, you do not need to relive what happened then. You simply need to write them down.

Extending your memory into your teen years, think about the types of foods you ate. Were there certain foods that you turned to when you were upset? Did one particular food make you feel safe? Loved? Popular? Among your friends, in what, if any, "food rituals" did you participate? For example, did you regularly hang out at the local pizza parlor every night? Or was the local ice cream shop your favorite dating spot? Whatever it was, write it down.

Moving into your adult years, think about the foods that were important to you then and still are today. Is there one food that you couldn't imagine living without? Do you regularly eat a certain food, sometimes to excess? Or is it absolutely mandatory that you eat a particular food every week, or even every day? If so, write the foods down. Make a list of those foods that you feel passionately about. Once again, it may be a good idea to take a break to give your subconscious some time to think about these questions.

After your break, go back over everything you have written. You are looking for patterns. Is there one food or even several that stand out? Do you constantly reach for a certain food when things seem difficult? Remember to read over everything you've written. It may be necessary to read through your writing a few times to notice the patterns. If you can't seem to find any patterns involving the same food, think about the types of food—high in sugar, salty or savory, crunchy items, etc. Whatever it is, simply write it down.

Now, for the next few days, try to notice your interaction with the foods you wrote down. When, if at all, do you find yourself eating these foods? If you're not eating them, do you find yourself thinking about them or planning to get them? Remember, this is not about judging yourself. You are investigating your eating habits, not condemning them. Not only is negativity extremely unhelpful at this point, it is unnecessary. If you seem to be spending a lot of time thinking negative things about yourself and/or your eating habits, try to remember the story about Adam and Eve. You are simply the product of your environment. Many situations and things made up the person you are today. Perhaps you are even unaware of the impact some of these events had on your life. That's why it is so important for you to simply become aware of what's happening. Judging it will only stand in the way of your investigation.

As you're noticing your interaction with the foods mentioned in your writing, try to notice how or if your child is involved with those foods as well. How easy this is will depend on the age of your child. If your child is in pre- or elementary school, you will probably have a lot more input into his or her meals than you would a child in high school. No matter what the age of your child, do not let him or her know what you are doing yet. Simply observe your child's eating habits without any additional comments. You may find it helpful to take notes about the things your child eats as well.

For instance, does your child insist on one particular food item for breakfast every day? If so, write it down. Are there certain food rules that your child follows every day—eating three candies at a time, having a cookie immediately upon arriving home from school, only eating green food, etc.? Whatever your child's food rituals are, simply write them down. You should plan to do this for several consecutive days. While recording your child's food on a "normal" day will be most helpful, during times that he or she is sick, you will still learn something. Just be sure to note the day or days of sickness so that you can compare them to the healthy days.

If you've been diligent about answering the questions and recording both your and your child's eating habits, you should have quite a bit of information to review. Your first step should be to compare your child's eating habits list to your own. What similarities do you find? What differences? Remember to also notice the eating times and situations. For example, does your child seem to need a snack around the same time that you do? Or does most of his or her eating (or overeating) take place at a certain time? Whatever you notice, write it down.

After you've done the comparison, look at the differences between the two. What does your child eat that you don't or won't? What (or when) do you eat that your child won't? Is there a certain time each day that both of you snack and/or overeat? Again, write down any patterns you discover. If you are raising your child with a partner, you may also take note of his or her eating habits as well by answering some of the previously mentioned questions and noting similar behaviors. Similarly, if you have more than one child—even if the other child isn't overweight—you may want to write down his or her eating behaviors, too. This is not to compare the children to each other but to create a picture of the household eating habits; therefore, if there are other members of the family and/or friends who live with you, take note of their eating habits as well.

By now, you're probably sick of writing. Even though it may seem tedious, there is a great need for you to have an accurate picture of the eating habits present in the household. Sometimes it's easy to miss certain activities simply because they are part of our normal lives. For instance, many overweight people drastically misrepresent the amounts of food they eat. Is this because they are lying? No. As addiction expert Abraham J. Twerski, MD points out in his book *Addictive Thinking*, "Denial . . . [is an] unconscious mechanism. . . often [a] gross distortion of truth, [yet true] to the addict." In other words, misrepresenting eating behaviors or amounts of food eaten is not a conscious decision, therefore, taking notes helps to break through any denial that may be present.

While you are taking notes about the household eating habits, it may be a good idea to also notice the level of physical activity that occurs. For instance, does your child come home from school and spend hours on the computer or watching television? Or, is he or she involved with a sports team or after-school activity? On weekends, does your family participate mostly in sedentary activities (watching movies, playing board games, reading) or physical events (bicycle riding, swimming, walking)? Again, be careful not to judge your family here. Just write.

When you've done this over a period of time, you have a pretty accurate picture of the eating habits and behaviors in your child's life. Putting it all together, what sort of conclusions can you reach? Does your child spend much of his or her free time eating high-calorie foods and participating in sedentary activities? Or is your child active yet overeating regularly? Do your child's eating habits reflect your own and/or your partner's? Did you notice whether or not there is great importance put on food in your household? Or did you recognize any of the behaviors described in the previous chapter?

For instance, after watching, writing, and thinking about some of the observations in this chapter, one mother came to the conclusion that she used food as a "common ground" for her and her child. Baking (and overeating) cookies had become a holiday event that they both looked forward to. Did you find something similar? Or did you find another way that food is used in your household? Do you or your children eat when under stress? Either way, it's important that you identify these patterns.

Remember, all you are being asked to do is identify the patterns. At this point in time, it would be self-defeating to try and change everything all at once. As you will come to see in the following chapter, dramatic changes such as these take time and patience. You cannot simply rush into changing a lifetime of eating and exercising behaviors based on the information in two chapters of a book. You will need more information and a solid plan to change things. More about this will be discussed in the following chapters.

For right now, I would like to share some of the ways that food was used in my life in the hopes that this will help you to identify similar patterns in your household.

Food was everything to me as a child. Even though I didn't know it at the time, I used food to nurture myself, to feel love, and as a way of relaxing. I can vividly remember coming home from school after being teased due to being overweight and eating potato chips and/or cookies. It never occurred to me that those were the very things that were making me fat. And even though I may have gone outside and played with others, there was not usually any type of physical activity involved. I enjoyed playing with Barbie dolls, a very sedentary activity to be sure.

Into my teen years, during which food played an even more important role, I often felt self-conscious, even ashamed of my body size. Rather than going out with others, I much preferred the safety of my own bedroom, with food to keep me company. I often planned my weekends around food and eating. As soon as I was able to drive, on Saturday nights, I would lie to my parents, telling them that I was going out with people from work. Instead, I would drive myself to a fast-food restaurant and order two double cheeseburgers with bacon, two large orders of french fries, and two diet sodas—that was so the server didn't think that I was the only one eating everything.

After getting my food, I would sit alone in my car in the parking lot, eating everything and watching everyone else have fun with their friends. To me, even though I didn't realize it at the time, food was my friend. It was easier to get along with and it never teased me.

Ballooning up to 328 pounds at my heaviest, I continued to use food in this way for many years, always planning my weekends to include food. When I was lonely, I ate. When I was sad or depressed, food was there. Even when I was happy, I still used food to express my emotions.

While I have also discovered that I have a physical addiction to food—more will be discussed about this in the chapter on eating disorders—my emotional dependence on food was just as devastating to my inner life as my physical addiction was to my body.

At 328 pounds, I hated myself and just about everyone else in my life. No one could do anything right, least of all me, and I barely made it through half a day without overeating. I felt humiliated because I couldn't control my weight and devastated by the effects. After twenty-three long years of suffering and hating myself, feeling as if I were an alien in the world, and putting my health in danger, I ended up in a food addiction treatment center for six weeks in order to figure out how to manage my life without using food.

While not everyone who uses food to nurture him- or herself or to celebrate ends up weighing 328 pounds, it is important for you to realize that without help, your child, too, may end up there. Helping your child to manage his or her feelings without using food is a serious matter that needs attention. Without this help, your child could very easily end up where I was or even worse-off. I know of one person whose top weight was just shy of 1,000 pounds. This person, who has since lost approximately 400 pounds, was near death and hated himself. The results of not learning to put food in its place are severe, even deadly.

Think about how many people get dangerous stomach bypass surgery. Though this may be beneficial in rare cases, most of these situations can be managed by learning what should have been taught during childhood—living a life where food is in its place. Personally, I know of two people, neither of whom was extremely overweight, who died from complications related to this surgery. Had these people learned the lessons you are about to, their lives could have been dramatically different.

Even though it is too late for these two people, your child has a chance. His or her habits can be changed. Your child can learn to de-emphasize food and live a life filled with healthy rather than destructive habits. So where do you begin? You may not like the answer.

It begins with you.

Though this may seem contrary to the message about not blaming yourself, it is not. While you are not to blame for your child's eating habits, you do serve as an example, both positive and negative. You are the single most important role model in your child's life. That means you will need to de-emphasize food in your life as well.

To begin, re-examine all of the writing you just did about your eating habits. If you decided to skip over that exercise, don't. Go back and do it. Though you may tell yourself that you can do it from memory, it will not work as well. There is no substituting the power of seeing a list of your eating habits written down in front of you. Without this list, you and your child will not receive the information necessary to fully change your eating habits. Think for a second about how many people lose weight yet regularly gain it back. Some experts put the success rate at as low as 2 percent for people who are able to keep off their lost weight for five years or more. Obviously, Americans are missing something in their weight-loss efforts and that "something" has been passed on to their children. The results you get from these exercises will be directly proportional to the efforts you put into these procedures.

Turning back to your writing, take a few minutes to study your eating habits. Where is there room for improvement? Are you overeating at certain times of the day and/or night? Even if you are sure that your child is asleep during your eating time, is it possible that he or she is aware of your actions? Without much effort, one of the most important things that you can do is to limit the amount of "junk" and fast food in your household. While you shouldn't attempt to immediately change your child's eating behaviors after rereading your lists, you can make a decision to omit or reduce the amount of junk food in your house.

If, for example, you usually buy three bags of cookies a month, buy only two and replace the third bag with some nonfat yogurt as a healthy alternative. If your child asks, you can simply say that you are trying to eat healthier. Do not, however, mention changing his or her habits. For reasons that will be discussed later, your child may rebel and may even become angry enough to seek out high-calorie food outside of the house. For right now, until you've read more, simply keep any discussion about a change in eating habits confined to you and your life.

Your child will need a chance to make up his or her own mind. This is true even in the case of a younger child.

After you have found a few areas where you could improve in your eating habits, begin to implement them. For instance, if you've decided to switch to low-fat instead of whole milk, you will be able to buy the new milk over the next day or two. But if you've decided to eat grilled chicken rather than the regular dinner of pizza on Sunday and it's only Monday, there is no need to mention this to your child tonight. Doing so may add to the importance your child places on food. When Sunday comes around, you can simply say that as part of your healthy eating plan, you have decided to try new and healthier foods on Sundays. It is important that you are nonchalant about this. Do not make a big deal or offer sympathy to your family. Simply say that cutting back on pizza is better for your health and that you would prefer not to eat it every Sunday. If your child is older and says that he or she will go out to get it, at this point, simply agree.

Remember, you do not want to become the food police for your child. Your goal here is to teach your child to make his or her own healthy choices. You will do this by the example that you set rather than through threats or intimidation. More specific tips will be presented in the following chapters; but for right now, the most important thing is that you not force your child into changing his or her eating habits. Simply concentrate on your own for right now. Eat and serve healthier meals without expressing distaste or anger about the food you are eating or your child's resistance to it.

It's also vital that you don't expect your child to change his or her eating habits overnight. In fact, in the beginning of your attempts to eat healthy, your child may eat more junk and fast food than before as a means of acting out his or her disappointment at being shut off from these foods at home. Though your first reaction may be to yell, criticize, or try to control your child's eating habits, resist the urge to do so. These behaviors will only serve to isolate and tempt your child. Think for a second what it was like when you were a child and your parents told you not to do something. Didn't it make you want to do whatever it was twice as much? And, given the first opportunity, didn't you go and do it? Do you honestly think that it will be any different for your child?

Even though the idea of simply standing by and watching your child eat more than he or she did before may be unappealing, it is necessary that your child be given freedom to explore healthy eating options. Try to relate it to when your child was learning to walk. If you had swooped in every time he or she stumbled, what would have happened? Children learn that a fall is not the end of the world and soon accept that if they persist in their efforts, the reward will be mastery of a new skill. While the attainment of developmental milestones differs from the establishment of habits, the idea is the same. Your child needs to learn to "fall" before succeeding. Your job is to let that happen, as difficult as it may be, and to continue with your own healthy eating behaviors.

Getting back to the title of this chapter, it begins with you. As you already know, eating behaviors are passed down from generation to generation. Even though this idea about examining family behaviors has been used to examine unhealthy eating behaviors, the concept works equally as well with healthy habits. In other words, you have the power to break the unhealthy eating cycle that has been passed down through your family. If you've always "hated" vegetables, consider serving different vegetables or cooking them in a different way to make them more appealing. For instance, using nonstick cooking spray to sauté onions and mushrooms together may seem less like the traditional broccoli you may have hated as a child but will serve as a healthy side dish.

In order to change both your habits and your child's, you will need to find creative ways to make healthy food appealing. To begin, make a list of the vegetables that you like or, at the very least, are able to tolerate. Then begin searching in cookbooks and/or on the Internet for recipes that seem appealing. Remember that in many cases you will need to make substitutions to make the dish healthy. Putting high-fat cheese sauce on broccoli is just as "dangerous" as eating a candy bar. To make your dishes healthy, try to stick to low-fat dressings such as tomato sauce, salsa, soy sauce, mustard, horseradish sauce, or lemon juice. Experiment by adding herbs and spices to enhance the flavor even further.

Though it may take a little time and some creativity, if you are persistent, you will be able to find at least one or two vegetable dishes that you and, eventually, your child will eat, perhaps even enjoy. When you do serve something new, simply put the dish on the table and let your child decide whether or not he or she will eat it. Make no comment either way. Do not offer praise and do not scold your child. Remember, you are trying to put food in its proper place in your child's life. Offering excessive praise for healthy eating puts undue importance on food, in the same way that scolding over unhealthy eating habits does. Simply put the healthy food on the dinner table and let your child make his or her decision.

Be sure to eat the food yourself, however. And if things don't go well, keep on trying. You may have to serve the dish a few times before your child comes around—and be prepared to accept that there may be some things that he or she will never eat. That's okay because if you are doing as suggested, all of the options on the dinner table will be healthy. A hungry child is bound to eat at least one of the options offered. The important thing here is to be consistent in your healthy eating behaviors. Do not offer healthy food one night and unhealthy food the next. This will simply confuse your child. In order to be successful, you will need to change your lifestyle permanently. Instead of viewing this as a diet that will end in a month or two, try using the "one- day-at-a-time" approach.

You are choosing to eat healthy for the rest of your life—but you are doing it one day at a time. In this way you can teach your child healthy eating habits that will last a lifetime.

Even though this may seem overwhelming at this point, remember that you don't have to change everything all at once nor do you have to figure out a lifetime of dinner menus today. Simply try to think about the next meal rather than the entire week or month. While you will need to plan ahead to grocery shop, you do not need to figure everything out right now. Try to make it through the next twenty-four hours only. Don't think about all of the events you have coming up. For now, just focus on today. Anything is manageable for twenty-four hours, while planning a whole lifetime at once is completely overwhelming. It's all a matter of how you think about it, and the choice is yours.

If you're still unclear about some of the ideas presented here, keep on reading. In the next chapter you will read about the role food should be playing in your child's life. In the following chapter, you will discover ways of managing life without using food to deal with emotional events. And in Chapter Five, you will discover ways of changing the harmful patterns that are present in your family. Until then, simply make an effort each day to introduce one healthy eating pattern into your child's life and accept that whatever he or she does with that is out of your control. Your actions, however, are not. Your child's healthy eating habits begin with you. It's important that you remember this as you continue reading.

Things to Remember

1. Don't try to do every suggestion all at once.
2. Small consistent steps are more effective than larger sporadic ones.
3. Serve as a role model for your child with your own eating habits.
4. Clear the house of all food you do not want your child to eat.
5. Do not try to control your child's eating patterns (unless, of course, he or she is very young). Instead, offer several healthy choices.
6. Though you may feel guilty, do not give in to this feeling.
7. Persistence is important. You are breaking habits that have been in place for a while.
8. Be creative in your cooking but don't put high-calorie "toppings" on healthy items.
9. Stay strong. Your child will try to coax you into giving him or her the food he or she is used to.
10. You are the single most important role model in your child's life.

CHAPTER THREE

⚜

WHAT FOOD ISN'T

FOOD MANUFACTURERS HAVE LONG MADE REMARKABLE efforts to market foods directly to children. Even more remarkable is the fact that these marketing efforts have been going on with little regulation for years. Think for a moment about all of the food icons throughout history created by manufacturers solely to sell food. We've had a dancing Carmen Miranda lookalike advertising the benefits of bananas (at least they're healthy); a squishy, Gingerbread-Man-like character nicknamed "Poppin' Fresh" (ironically, since he advertises refrigerated dough products); and a talking tiger on two legs who pronounces sweetened breakfast cereal to be "G-r-r-e-e-a-a-t!" to name just a few.

In addition to these manufacturer-created food icons, there are those already popular cultural icons used to promote specific foods. Think, for instance, about a cartoon mischief-maker's affinity for a certain candy bar, upon which no one had better "lay a finger." Baby-like symbols of innocence with silly sounding names are sponsored by fast-food burger chains. The stone age and the space age each have their own cartoons and those cartoon characters are used to advertise breakfast cereals. Even old, established, tablet-shaped, multi-character candy dispensers keep up with the times, introducing new dispensers tied to movie blockbusters and cultural icons each season.

Though these are only a few examples, there are many more to prove exactly how ingrained marketing food to children is in American society. Think for a second about your own childhood. While the marketing efforts were probably not as flashy or sophisticated as they are today, food advertisements and marketing efforts were still very visible. The problem is that most people aren't aware of and are only just beginning to learn to identify them. Remember the caramel-coated popcorn associated with the All-American pastime, baseball? What was the best part of eating that sweetened popcorn and peanut confection? Was it the prize inside? Or, perhaps it was the decoder ring in your sugary breakfast cereal that you looked forward to. Either way, these early efforts represent food manufacturers' attempts to make food fun and interesting for children. And the problem has only gotten worse and continues to worsen.

Numerous studies and articles have emerged in recent years, indicating that the food and beverage industry in the US has children and adolescents in its sights, targeting them as a major market force. Children and adolescents have become the focus of intense, sophisticated, food marketing and advertising efforts, not only because of their present-day purchasing influence, but also as future adult consumers.

Various methods, techniques, and channels are used to reach youngsters, beginning when they are toddlers, to promote brand-building and to influence purchasing behavior around food. These include television advertising, in-school marketing, product placements, kids clubs, the Internet, including social media, toys and products with brand logos, and youth-targeted promotions, such as cross-selling and tie-ins. And of course, most foods marketed to children are predominantly high in sugar and fat, and as such are inconsistent with national dietary recommendations.

Before discussing the health implications of marketing food to children, it is important to understand the full scope of the problem.

The Rudd Center for Food Policy and Obesity at Yale University, a nonprofit research and public policy organization dedicated to improving the world's diet, preventing obesity and reducing weight stigma has as one of its core research initiatives the marketing of food to youths. At the organization's website, (http://fastfoodmarketing.org), there are many fast-food facts. Among those listed are:

- The fast-food industry spent more than $4.2 billion dollars in 2009 on TV advertising and other media.
- The average preschooler (2–5 years) saw 2.8 TV ads per day for fast food; children (6–11 years) saw 3.5; and teens (12–17 years) saw 4.7.
- Young people's exposure to fast-food TV ads has increased. Compared to 2003, preschoolers viewed 21 percent more fast-food ads in 2009, children viewed 34 percent more, and teens viewed 39 percent more.
- Although McDonald's and Burger King have pledged to improve food marketing to children, they increased their volume of TV advertising from 2007 to 2009. Preschoolers saw 21 percent more ads for McDonald's and 9 percent more for Burger King, and children viewed 26 percent more ads for McDonald's and 10 percent more for Burger King.
- Even though McDonald's and Burger King only showed their "better-for-you" foods in child-targeted marketing, their ads

did not encourage consumption of these healthier choices. Instead, child-targeted ads focused on toy giveaways and building brand loyalty.

- Children saw more than child-targeted ads. More than 60 percent of fast-food ads viewed by preschoolers and children promoted fast-food items other than kids' meals.

The takeaway from all this is that fast-food marketing is ubiquitous and persistent.

According to one expert, in a given year, Americans will spend over $110 billion on fast food—more than they'll spend on movies, books, magazines, newspapers, videos, and recorded music combined.

The obesity rate among preschoolers has doubled in the past thirty years. Oddly the annual cost of the nation's obesity epidemic—about $168 billion, as calculated by researchers at Emory University—is the same amount of money Americans spent on fast food in a year.

Think for a minute about the many other food promotions directed at children. How many can you name? How many is your child exposed to? Even more important, how many influence your child? Take a second to look around your child's room. Is it filled with promotional items from food manufacturers? How many times during the week does your child ask you to buy a food item? Is this the direct result of the slick marketing efforts of food manufacturers? It may help for you to make a list of the food items your child requests over the next week. While doing this, take note of the commercials or advertisements your child has been exposed to. Does the latest movie character appear on the candy your child requests? Or is the comic book character strategically placed on the potato chip package your child begs for?

Whatever it is, write it down without trying to analyze it. Then, when the week is over, take a good look at the list. Are the food items your child requests associated with fun and/or excitement? Does use of these food items seem to "guarantee" that your child will experience acceptance, love, adoration, and/or attention? One of the most obvious ways food manufacturers convey the promise of adoration or acceptance is to associate their products with young celebrities. This is especially true of soda companies. Pop princesses and the most popular "boy band" members promote sugary, fizzy, cola drinks; and soda producers themselves sponsor youth-oriented "talent" and award shows that create new "stars" for youngsters to emulate and adore.

Co-sponsorships such as this associate high-calorie food and drinks with the promise of achieving celebrity status. For awkward, insecure children and teens, the promise of fan adulation, money, and power can be strong. This, combined with the photographically altered images of stars "having fun" and seemingly being free to do as they please, can be a powerful motivator for children and/or teens to eat or drink large quantities of the items promoted by these celebrities. For children and teens raised in a "more-is-better" culture like ours, it is not difficult to see how the so-called positive attributes of being a celebrity can be associated with eating and/or drinking certain items. The reasoning may go something like this—if Starlet X drinks Buzz Cola and everyone loves her, then maybe if I drink a lot of Buzz Cola, I will be popular, too. Even though you know this isn't true, to a child and/or teen it may seem perfectly logical—in fact, it's unlikely there will be reasoning involved at all, as this process will most likely take place on a subconscious level, of which he or she is not even aware.

The added danger with this sort of thinking is that the items promoted by these celebrities and believed to be magical by children and teens are usually high in sugar and calories, thus contributing to an already high obesity rate. Think for a second about how many young celebrities or cartoon characters you have seen promoting healthy foods. Does your child's favorite superhero promote carrots, or any other vegetable, for that matter? Has today's hot singing sensation ever promoted fruit? The answer to these questions is a big "no." Even the mere suggestion of this is almost laughable. This by itself should tell you something—celebrities, superheroes, cartoon icons, and singing sensations almost always promote high-calorie food items, all but ignoring healthy products.

In addition to this, the items promoted by these celebrities cannot be used to excess if the flawless skin and thin bodies necessary for stardom are to be achieved. In other words, even though celebrities promote high-calorie items, it is fair to assume that they don't overindulge or, perhaps, ever indulge in them on a regular basis. Once again, promotions such as these couple food with feelings of excitement and acceptance rather than encourage children to eat to nourish their bodies. In order to put this into perspective, it is important to examine the scope of the problem. To begin, let's consider the amount of money food manufacturers regularly spend on promoting high-calorie foods to your child.

Fast-food advertising budgets in the United States have grown exponentially since the early days of television, and the ads get more pervasive all the time. You are probably all too familiar with the fairly recent phenomenon of "stealth" advertising—ads disguised as something else or placed where you least expect to encounter an ad. Included in this form of advertising is the practice called "product placement," wherein manufacturers pay large sums of money to get their brands shown in films, sometimes even getting scripts rewritten to showcase the product. Other forms of stealth advertising include corporate-sponsored events. Just about every cultural event has a corporate sponsor—those sponsors have a lot of influence over their beneficiaries.

According to their own figures, at least a billion dollars a year is spent by just one fast-food chain to persuade families to visit a bizarre-looking clown's playground and while there, purchase a thousand calories for a mere $2.50. Please think about that dollar amount just one chain spends yearly on advertising. The number is "at least a billion dollars." A billion dollars! Imagine how much exposure that much money gets a company. Now couple this with the fact that in the majority of the ads presented, food is not the only thing being sold. It's an experience—a lifestyle if you will.

According to the Rudd Center, children as young as two years old are targeted on the website of a fast-food giant's mascot. Both of the top two chains have websites with virtual worlds and "advergames." The Rudd Center further notes that one of these sites got 365,000 unique child visitors and 294,000 unique teen visitors on average *each month* in 2009. That's a very smart strategy if they're trying to build a long-term relationship.

Preschool and school-aged children are both the subjects and the targets of these ads, and an infant is actually featured in one of the top company's most recent commercials. The ad features a young father playing with his gurgling baby. "There will be a first step, a first word, and, of course, a first french fry," says the warm voice of a young woman on the soundtrack. As the theme song ends, the image on screen fades to a french fry that curves into the shape of a smile.

Though the company denies directly targeting children, you can certainly judge for yourself what the message is here: it's perfectly acceptable to start kids on these unhealthy foods while they are still in high chairs. This message has repercussions that can be tragic.

Taking this a step further, advertisers have even invaded

schools. Channel One, a news program in middle and high schools, is currently in 8,000 schools and reaches approximately six million students nationwide. At a time when shrinking budgets are contributing to increased class size and loss of instructional time, I believe that the estimated one full day per year lost to Channel One's commercials is unconscionable. And, of course, many of those commercials are for the types of foods that are unhealthy.

Consider that most high schools, many middle schools, and almost half of all elementary schools contain vending machines and/or stores that students can freely access. Despite the fact that schools receiving funding from the USDA are required to meet that organization's nutritional guidelines for foods they serve as lunches, among the 88 percent that do participate, there are loopholes. Schools must offer lunches that contain no more than thirty percent of calories from fat, but this requirement only applies to the official school lunch. Foods purchased *a la carte* from menus are exempt, and about sixty percent of elementary schools and eighty-four percent of high schools offer *a la carte* foods. And only a little more than half of students buy official school lunches to begin with.

In addition to this, schools receive large amounts of money for making exclusive deals with soft drink manufacturers. Despite the fact that these items can't be sold during breakfast and lunch periods, schools have found a way to increase sales. "They [schools] can also sell these foods in other areas of the campus—even right outside the cafeteria door—any time they want. And although schools can't sell soda in cafeterias during lunch, they can give it away," says [Director of Nutrition Policy at the Center for Science in the Public Interest Margo] Wootan. "[It's] a way to entice kids to eat in the school meals program," she explains.

Add to this the fact that $750 million is spent annually to sell snacks and processed foods in schools. "Companies like Coca-Cola and Pepsi offer schools hundreds of thousands of dollars a year in exchange for exclusive vending machine contracts. And financially pinched schools can't resist. This is such an incredibly bad idea, because the school enters into a contract that puts them in the position of encouraging kids to drink more soda so that they can make more money. They often get bonuses if kids drink more," says Wootan.

Additionally, consider that inside and outside of schools, food manufacturers are constantly thinking of new ways to market food to children while parents are becoming less involved in eating choices, and you have some idea of the growing problem. In a study published in the Canadian publication, the *Journal of Paediatrics & Child Health* in November 2011, Lana Hebden and her colleagues studied persuasive marketing techniques directed at children in Sydney, Australia. The researchers concluded that the marketing techniques most prominent in unhealthy food advertisements were "palatability (54 percent of unhealthy food advertisements), convenience (52 percent), fantasy/imagination (28 percent), fun/happiness (17 percent), and cartoon characters (9 percent)." While this study was conducted in Sydney, it is safe to assume that the results would be similar in the US.

It only makes sense that palatability or good taste would be a selling point in targeting children, as is convenience. The last three, fantasy/imagination, fun/happiness, and cartoon characters, however, are a problem. Consider for a second that these three categories combined represent 54 percent of the marketing techniques used. This means that areas such as fantasy and fun, which do not have anything to do with providing nutrition for your child's body, are being used to promote unhealthy foods.

Add to this the previous discussion about cartoon characters and you have a pretty good idea of how much "fun" your children are expecting from unhealthy foods. An April 2010 study published in *Public Health Nutrition*, a journal for academic researchers, found that cross-promotions involving third-party characters accounted for 71 percent of the products directed at children. Fifty-seven percent of these were directed at children under twelve.

The sheer volume of advertising to which children are exposed makes the picture even more dire. Most experts agree that children see about 40,000 commercials each year, though some put the number much higher. Repeated exposures to ads increase their effectiveness. Very young children don't distinguish between a commercial and television programming. And children under eight aren't able to understand that ads are created to convince people to buy products. Think about some of the toys your children play with.

Many of these toys are actually foods. Toy helicopters come replete with replaceable canisters filled with candy-coated chocolate candies. Spinning lollipops that fit into a battery-operated handle and linked to media hits such as Spider-Man, Powerpuff Girls, and Batman are popular; some even vibrate and make sounds when you push a button. Such products are turning play—the birthright of every child—into a health issue.

Seemingly innocent toys actually contribute to a deadly problem—childhood obesity. Even though it seems harmless enough to have a fast-food fashion doll or a candy-filled helicopter, think for a second about the hidden messages your child is getting by associating food with playtime. Playing is something children do to have fun. When food-related products are brought into that fun time, children begin to associate food and eating with having fun and playing. There are two problems with this.

The first, and most obvious, is that by playing with food, children have amped up the very real emotion of happiness inherent to the process of having fun. Children who use food in their playtime come to associate positive feelings with food, thus setting up what could be a lifelong pattern of expecting food to fulfill emotional, instead of merely nutritional, needs. Remember the examples at the beginning of this book? Each and every one— with the possible exception of the baby crying—had a beginning. And that beginning could very well have been during playtime with toys that involve food. These toys set up a pattern of associating food with fun and play. This being so, think about how an elementary school student, an adolescent, or a teenager wanting to have fun will go about that. Where do you think they will turn? Though admittedly this may happen on an unconscious level, by the time a child has grown into a teenager, a clear pattern is established. Food will ALWAYS equal fun to this young adult who will undoubtedly turn into an overweight adult.

Another danger of using food during playtime is it makes those items more special than other foods. And since most of the foods being promoted are high in calories and fat, children will come to believe that items high in calories and fat are more desirable than healthy ones. Not only will this establish what could be a lifelong pattern but children who grow into teens will come to prefer certain foods for reasons that may have nothing to do with taste. While it is hard to deny that high-calorie foods generally taste better, why would a parent want that message reinforced during playtime? The mere fact that you are reading this book shows that you would not.

Perhaps one of the greatest challenges of learning to help your child live a healthy life is the fact that to be most effective, you will need to rethink some of those things that you and the rest of society may have taken for granted. In addition to the food and play in examples presented above, you may want to consider some other habits or rituals that society and, maybe even your family, participate in regularly. Though some of them have been previously mentioned, it bears repeating as these rituals are so ingrained in American culture. Following is a list of ways in which food is used for purposes other than for nourishment.

Cake is eaten on one's birthday. Ice cream is served at countless children's parties. Chocolate is given at Valentine's Day. Cookies are baked for holidays. Candy canes are given during Christmas. Baskets filled with candy are given at Easter. Barbecues mark Memorial, Independence, and Labor Days. Anniversaries are celebrated with special dinners. Carnivals and State Fairs are filled with cotton candy, fried foods, and chocolate. Movie theater lobbies have refreshment stands with buckets full of popcorn. Nearly every public beach has an ice cream stand. And large portions of most malls are devoted to mammoth food courts.

Fast-food restaurants are open just about around the clock, and dining out has become an adventure for many. Upscale restaurants boast phenomenal views or elaborate themes and even slow-moving floors to provide 180-degree views. Exorbitantly priced meals have become status symbols. Cooking shows regularly fill television airwaves, with an entire channel devoted specifically to food. Chefs are given celebrity status and cooking programs are now viewed for their entertainment value. Warehouse stores sell food items in gargantuan quantities while "super-sizing" is becoming (has become) an American way of life.

Entire sections of bookstores are devoted to cookbooks, and several cooking magazines boast circulations in the millions. A large hot dog-shaped car tours the country, oftentimes stopping at schools or offering children the chance to appear in national commercials. Just about every movie released for children today has a food tie-in and, in some cases, specialized candy items for children to eat. Talking candies and food icons regularly make appearances at theme parks, shopping malls, and even public libraries; celebrities vigorously promote high-calorie food items on their shows and at their concerts. Children who aren't allowed to freely eat cookies and candy are viewed as deprived; grocery store fliers are filled with specially priced food items targeted to children. Just about every school or church event is followed, if not dominated, by a period of eating—church picnics, cookie time, ice cream socials, etc.

Though this list may seem exhaustive, it is not. There are many other events in American culture that revolve around or involve food. And though they may seem harmless due to the familiarity of the practices, it's important to remember that there is great danger in using food for anything besides the nourishment for which it is intended. If drugs were offered to children in the amounts and quantities that food is at these festivities, no parent would expose a child to these events, any more than he or she would bring a child to a crack house. The mere thought of this is absurd!

Yet, let's consider the analogy for a second longer. We understand that drugs are harmful and can kill children, but what about food? Well, the obesity rate in children has doubled over the past few decades, and children are developing diabetes at a much younger and more severe rate. More Americans than ever are overweight and more than 400,000 deaths each year are related to excess weight and/or lack of physical activity, according to the CDC. The National Institute of Health estimates that the total cost for obesity-related diseases is nearly $100 billion per year. Approximately eight million Americans join diet programs every year. Over 98 percent of all Americans who begin diets regain the weight back plus more within five years.

It is important to note that some of these studies' statistics have been challenged or are thought to be exaggerated. Even if this is true (there has been no across-the-board consensus), there seems to be a consensus that more than 100,000 people succumb to obesity-related deaths each year, though many experts put the number much higher.

Does it seem extreme to characterize food as "dangerous" and even "deadly?" We usually reserve such descriptions for things like cigarettes, alcohol, or other drugs. But to a person who is already at risk because of obesity, or who may be addicted to food, such a characterization is not extreme. Used for its legitimate purpose, food is beneficial and nourishing; but it can be as dangerous as any other substance of abuse to a person who is overweight or obese or addicted to it. And although the stigma of addiction has yet to be completely eradicated, it can still be easier to find genuine help for addiction than for obesity, for which the touted solutions frequently turn out to be scams or, at the very least, misleading or false information.

Another thing to keep remembering is that you can't—nor should you try to—change everything at once. For example, it would be impossible to change the way society, or even your child's school, encourages eating. To try to tackle such an entrenched aspect of American culture would only cause frustration for you and your child. Instead, concentrate on what is within your control—your household environment.

As the adult, you are the one who will make food-purchasing choices and that's where your greatest progress can be made. By making high-calorie items unavailable in your home, you have already made important progress in helping your child. Even though you may not like some of the information presented, now that you have read this far, please don't stop or feel overwhelmed by the task before you. Feeling uncomfortable about bucking society's eating practices is only natural. Remember, many of the traditions and activities mentioned in this chapter are part of most people's daily lives. There is no shame in admitting that you and your family participate in some of the activities mentioned.

This book is not about condemning you or your child. Rather, the idea is to make you aware of potential danger areas that are currently affecting your child's life. Some of these you may choose to change and some you may not; but, at least with the knowledge presented here, your choice will be based on your family and your family's needs and not on habits or customs that have never been investigated. In other words, the most powerful weapon you have in the battle against emotional overeating and childhood obesity is knowledge. The more you know, the better chance your child has of living a healthy life. So please continue reading.

Things to Remember

1. Advertisers are using many different methods to encourage children to eat unhealthy food.

2. Food is not about having fun, but many advertising campaigns include creating games (fun) that involve unhealthy foods so children will want to eat them.

3. The obesity rate among children is growing quickly. Some experts estimate that it has tripled in the past thirty years.

4. It isn't just advertisements that are contributing to the obesity epidemic. Vending machines or stores that students can freely access are included in most all high schools, many middle schools, and almost half of all elementary schools.

5. In order to help your child, you may need to rethink many things, including the ways he or she plays.

6. The National Institute of Health estimates that the total cost

for obesity-related diseases is nearly $100 billion per year. Approximately eight million Americans join diet programs every year.

7. Food is beneficial and nourishing, but if used improperly, such as to reward behavior, dangerous patterns may develop that could result in addiction to food.

8. Do not try to make drastic changes all at once. You've heard the saying, "Slow and steady wins the race?" Slow, steady, and consistent effort works much better than intense efforts that may be inconsistent.

CHAPTER FOUR

❦

WHAT FOOD IS

HOW MANY TIMES HAVE YOU BEEN CONFUSED by the nutritional information that you've read? How often have you given up trying simply because you couldn't figure out what was best for your child?

If these things have happened to you, don't worry. You aren't alone. According to some experts, confusing the public is one of the four methods food manufacturers use to sell more food. In addition to manufacturing foods that appeal to the public's taste preferences for sweetness, fat, and salt, attempting to keep prices low while adding value, and offering great convenience by making eating fast, food companies try to keep the public confused as a means of increasing sales of their products.

Think for a second about the nutritional information you've read. Parenting magazines are filled with information about the latest health breakthroughs. Women's magazines regularly feature health and nutritional information, and television news programs discuss recent health innovations. And much of the information seems to contradict the "breakthroughs" of the recent past, leading to more confusion. Do calories count, or are carbs more important? How vital are vitamins? Can kids get all their protein if they don't eat meat? What is a parent to do?

For starters, don't forget that media outlets need to focus on breakthroughs and controversies in order to sell their products—magazines, broadcasts, and newspapers. The public tires of reading articles that simply reinforce the common wisdom, and they enjoy the excitement of controversy and argument instead. So it's no wonder that as each "new" nutritional "discovery" is trumpeted, adherents of the previous "breakthrough" are given "equal time" to defend their opinions—it sells newspapers. (It also confuses readers, but as long as the readers keep looking to the media for answers, the media will keep supplying them.) And on it goes.

Add to this the reality that food companies must satisfy shareholders by selling more and more of their products, which in turn fills the media with more and more advertising. It is no wonder we become confused by the avalanche of information—in articles *and* ads—that comes at us day after day.

Unfortunately, most people get the bulk of their nutrition advice, not from impartial sources, like a government agency, but from the food industry itself. As we have seen, this is hardly an unbiased source, and its agenda is often at odds with that of the consumers who wish to feed themselves and their families in a healthful manner.

Yet the basic truths have not changed. "Eat less fat and sugar. Smaller portions are better. Get more exercise. Eat more fruit and vegetables." Perhaps the problem is that such advice is so obvious that it's boring! So when looking to the media for nutritional advice, always "consider the source," and remember that research results are open to interpretation—if the people doing the interpreting are employed by the food companies, they may interpret the results in a way that satisfies their employers.

Putting all of this together, the message of this chapter is consistent with that of the entire book—food and eating are a means of nourishing your body. They are not meant to quell emotions, control anxiety, express love, or deliver fun. Food is simply a means of nourishing your child's body. Read that again and again if necessary—food is meant only for nourishment. Despite what food manufacturers may try to tell us, food is simply a means of nourishing your body. Period.

I write this in the hopes that the full extent of the problem will become clear through my own personal example. As I described earlier, by the time I was twenty-three, I weighed 328 pounds; but what you don't know is that despite the fact that I have lost nearly 150 pounds and kept it off for many years, I still live with many consequences of my obesity even today.

After years of overeating items high in processed sugar and flour, the brain chemicals in my body became altered, which resulted in a physical addiction to sugar and flour—an addiction similar to that experienced by any other addict. And as with any addict, to remain sane and free of the intense physical cravings for my substance, I need to abstain from eating food items containing sugar and flour. In addition, because of the emotional dependence on food that I developed, I need to weigh and measure every item that goes into my mouth—without exception. Even after twenty-three years in recovery, there are some times when I have difficulty determining correct portions; that's when it helps to have the tools of a program on which to rely.

All of this means that I cannot ever eat cake on my birthday; that I did not have even one bite of my wedding cake; that I will never be able to eat a piece of bread without making my body and my mind ill. If I take even one bite of a cookie, I may not ever stop overeating again. When I am extremely emotional or even sometimes when I'm not, I am unable to determine what a "normal" serving size of anything is. This is why I weigh and measure all of my food. Even when on vacation, I cannot overeat or eat food items with sugar or flour in them. I do not have ice cream in the summer or hot cocoa in the winter. Dessert is never an option and sometimes I abstain from certain functions because I choose not to have to deal with being around large amounts of food.

Physically, despite my weight loss and a rigorous exercise program, there are parts of my body that will never be a normal size. In order to have normal-sized arms and a flat stomach, I had to undergo a surgical procedure to remove the excess skin hanging from my upper arms and stomach area. Even with the surgery, I still have three large scars—one on each arm and across my stomach. My legs, however, are different. Even with my weight loss, my calves will never be a normal size. I will never be able to wear normal-sized boots or even some tapered pants. Dresses and ankle bracelets will only exaggerate my problem.

Despite all of this, I am one of the lucky ones, as for the past twenty-three years I have been able to maintain a substantial weight loss. As you already know, fewer than 5 percent of the people who go on diets each year manage to keep off the weight they lose for more than five years. And, though my method may seem extreme, after years of failed dieting attempts, I have finally found something that works for me and I am able to live a sane life. Before finding my current program, I thought constantly about food, but now these thoughts—this obsession—does not rule my life.

The point I am making here is that there are many devastating consequences to being overweight, other than simple aesthetics. As a child, I was teased mercilessly, ostracized during recess, and shunned publicly. As a teenager, I stayed home and ate rather than go out in public due to my body size. I never attended one high school dance, did not have a boyfriend at school, was not invited to the prom, and never participated in extracurricular activities. My idea of relaxation and fun was to sit at home reading and watching television while eating. I had no hobbies or personal interests besides eating, and I did not know how to communicate my distress to anyone.

By the time I was in my late teens, I was wearing big men's clothes, my feet ached due to the excess weight I carried, and I could barely walk up a flight of stairs without great effort. At least once I week, I was too overwhelmed by life and depressed to even get out of bed, missing school regularly. I had no professional or personal goals, only attending college because my father agreed to help me pay for a new car if I did. At college, I only did enough to get by, never fully committing to anything. The older I got, the worse my overeating became and the more miserable my life was.

At twenty-three, I was suicidal and desperate. I hated myself and I hated just about everyone in my life. I didn't enjoy anything, not even eating. Each morning I promised myself that I would begin a diet, only to overeat by noon. I considered myself to be weak-willed and beyond hope, many times wishing that I had the courage to kill myself so that my pain would end.

Even though my experience was extreme, it's vital that you are aware of the consequences that come from overeating. One of the reasons I developed a physical addiction to sugar and flour is because I ate so much of these substances that eventually my body developed a dependence on them. In other words, at some point in my life I could have stopped myself before I crossed the line into a full-blown addiction had I been aware. The key to this idea is in the last part of that sentence: *had I been aware.* I never even knew that it was possible to be addicted to sugar and flour, and I certainly never considered the emotional attachment I had to food. I simply looked at myself as someone who was too weak-willed to diet, never suspecting that I had a physical and emotional addiction to certain foods.

Since you've picked up this book, however, your awareness will help your child to live a healthy life. Just knowing that there are ways to help your child eat healthier is a big part of taking steps to make it better. Until I knew what my problem was, I certainly couldn't take steps to solve it or prevent it from progressing. Now that you are aware of the difficulties regarding food that your child faces, you have taken an important first step toward helping him or her.

Just how are you to go about helping? The first and most important thing to remember is that making changes such as the ones needed is not easy. Change is not easy nor is it pleasant. Think about the last time you had to make even a small change in your daily routine. How long did it take you to get used to it? How difficult did you find making the change? Did you eventually go back to the routine you were used to? If you stayed with the new routine, when did you finally become comfortable? Now imagine trying to change habits that were set in motion by your great-great-great-grandparents. Seems overwhelming, doesn't it?

The most significant thing that you need to take away from this chapter is the fact that though making changes is difficult, it is not impossible. Even though people in your life may be resistant, you need to remember what is at stake—your child's health. Because eating rituals are so firmly ingrained in society, your efforts will not go unchallenged by others. A characteristic of American society is instant gratification without regard to consequences. As an example, think for a second about how many convenience foods there are currently on the market. In some grocery stores, the frozen food aisles are larger than the entire produce department. And what types of foods fill these aisles? Ice cream? Pizza? Fried chicken? Pies? Chances are, you'll see them all.

Now, think about the bakery and packaged-foods aisles. Most of these products are designed to make life more convenient and food tastier for consumers. And this is accomplished by adding fat and sugar. Despite nutritional tables on packages listing serving sizes and calories, these items sell extremely well.

The instant gratification of good taste seems to be more important than the consequences of eating foods high in fat and calories. Many Americans spend a great deal of time talking about losing weight but relatively few put in the effort to take the steps necessary to accomplish this.

Even our media promote the idea of effortless weight loss—think of your favorite magazine. Is there a story about losing weight in the same issue as a section on dessert recipes? What about articles on Hollywood starlets in a seeming competition to return to their "pre-baby weight" as quickly as possible after giving birth? On the cover, do you find a picture of a cake right next to information about the latest weight-loss plan? Combining weight loss articles with dessert recipes is common practice for many magazines—these mixed messages are especially evident in publications directed at women. It seems magazine editors, at least, believe they can fool most of the readers most of the time, convincing them that they can have their cake and lose weight, too. No wonder Americans are so willing to believe it; it's right there in black and white!

The fact that most people seem to want the benefits of losing weight without making the sacrifices necessary to achieve weight loss may be the biggest hurdle when making changes in your family's eating habits. The mixed messages that have been delivered by our society allow people to continue to talk about losing weight without actually having to give up eating dessert items. Talking requires little effort, while developing healthy eating patterns takes a great deal of work. Persons without the same interest in your child's health that you have may discourage your efforts to change the status quo.

Think about the last holiday gathering you attended. How many times were you or your child urged to have "just one" cookie or other high-calorie item to celebrate the holiday? And did the person doing the urging join you? Or did someone remind you of how hard they worked at preparing a high-calorie dish in an attempt to get you to eat some? Was there guilt involved if you turned down this person's food? Take a second to think about the interactions regarding food at holiday gatherings. Is there one person who can be considered a "food pusher" much in the same way that drug dealers push their products? Consider this person's lifestyle for a second. Is he or she overweight or concerned about eating healthy? Does he or she regularly attempt to diet?

Think about this person's eating habits. If he or she is dieting, the food pushing may be an attempt to compensate for those things currently not being eaten. If there is no diet involved, he or she may simply be looking for someone to overeat with. Remember the old adage about misery loving company? Well, in the case of someone who is not dieting, he or she may be looking for "company" to justify the overeating. The thinking goes like this—*if so-and-so is eating three pieces of cake, then it must be okay for me, too.* If dieting *is* involved then he or she may be looking for an excuse to cheat—*if so-and-so can eat that, then why can't I?* Even though this person may not eat the food right then, he or she may be waiting to eat in private later. Either way, these are some of the kinds of challenges you may be faced with when you try to change your family's eating habits.

There are several ways to deal with resistance from family and friends. To begin, one of the best skills that you can learn while changing your family's eating habits is to say "no" without offering an explanation. Though this may seem rude, it is not. Despite what society may tell us, "no" is a complete sentence. There is no need to explain why you are refusing to eat certain high-calorie foods. Simply say, "no, thank you." If you are pressed, simply repeat your statement and move on to another topic of conversation. A firm and simple "no" will go a long way toward ending urgings from others to eat foods that will harm your family's health. If you offer an explanation, then you have opened yourself up for others to comment on your new way of eating or to try to talk you out of it.

For example, a conversation may go something like this:

"Would you like to try the cookies I baked yesterday?"

"No thanks. We're all trying to eat healthier."

"Oh, come on. Just one won't hurt. And it's a new recipe."

"No, we really need to watch what we eat."

"Oh, how many calories could one cookie have in it?"

"No, I'm worried about how heavy Sam is getting and I want us all to support him in losing weight."

"Are you telling me that you're never going to have a cookie again? How realistic is that?"

"No, but . . ."

"Here, just take a bite to try it. You don't even have to finish the whole thing."

At this point, you are probably so frustrated—even doubtful about the healthy choices you have made—that you may give in. Or maybe you are more resilient, but a little more urging will wear you down to the point at which you give in and try the cookie. Either way, you have eaten something that you didn't want to. Though this may not seem too serious, think about what happened during the conversation. Your friend not only urged you to eat but you engaged in a debate about your entire new lifestyle, making it easier for you to question what you are doing. The consequences of this can be very severe.

For instance, if you decide to eat the cookie, then it may be easier to have something else as well, which will eventually lead you back to your old way of life. While it may be easy to be angry at your friend, think for a second. Haven't you done the same thing in the past? Your friend is only doing what he or she has been trained by society to do— provide food as a means of showing affection.

It's important to remember that your refusal of the food is NOT a reflection on your feelings for the person offering it to you. Remember, food is simply a means of nourishing your body. It was never meant to be a way of expressing affection or friendship.

After you refuse your friend's offer of food, you may feel guilty. This is especially true if the refusal involves a relative. Because of the messages regularly created by advertisers, many people will take your refusal personally and may even be offended. What do you do about this? It's quite simple—let them have their feelings even if they are insulted. Eventually, they will get over it, but in the meantime you have made an important choice about the future of your family's health. And once the initial guilt is gone, you will be proud of yourself for taking such a firm stand.

While you are feeling guilty, however, it's vital that you don't use food to deal with these feelings. Though it may sound ridiculous, many people end up eating after such a confrontation to lessen the feelings of guilt. Be aware that after one of these interactions, you are most vulnerable to overeating. If you are like most people, you have at times used food in some way to nurture yourself; and when you're feeling guilty, you need nurturing. It only makes sense that food would be the first thing you would think of. But resist the urge and try to think of something else with which to nurture yourself instead.

This is actually another skill that will become invaluable during this transitional phase—learning to nurture yourself. It may be a good idea to make a list of activities that soothe you. Remember that anything involving food, with the exception of herbal tea or decaffeinated coffee, should not be on this list. Be careful not to include "sneaky" food activities such as baking cookies, looking at cookbooks, taking the children to a fast-food playland, watching television cooking shows, or playing with your food-related toys. These activities will only "feed" your guilt and make it difficult for you to continue with your healthy lifestyle.

If you find it difficult to make this list, this may be an indication of exactly how ingrained food and eating are in your life. Try to think about the activities that you enjoy. Does a long hot bath relax you? Would getting a manicure make you feel special? Will a little time in the garden lift your spirits? Or how about a walk by the beach? A drive in the country? A game of chess? An old movie? A horseback ride? Whatever it is, write it down. Try to think of as many things as you can. This way, if you are unable to complete your first choice, you will have additional options. Also coming up with two or three quick alternatives will help. For instance, taking three long deep breaths, praying, rubbing your neck, splashing water on your face, looking at a special picture or inspirational saying—any of these things can be accomplished in only a matter of minutes. This will be especially helpful when you are rushed.

Another necessary skill to develop when changing your lifestyle is to say what you mean. If you seem uncertain in your decisions and food choices, your children and the people in your life will use this as a way of trying to change your mind. Once you have refused to eat a certain food, it is important that you do not eat it later. If you do, your friends and family will find it difficult to believe that you are serious about your new way of life. Similarly, if you have refused one high-calorie dessert, do not reach for an equally fattening one minutes later. This will undermine your credibility and make others doubt you in the future when you refuse high-calorie items. Being consistent in your choices will make it easier for you in the future. In the same way that the people in your life are used to your eating certain things now, they will eventually become accustomed to your new way of life. Someday, though it may not seem possible now, there will even come a point when these people may even cease to ask if you want to eat high-calorie foods. This is when you will know that your new way of eating is firmly ingrained in your life.

So what do all of these new habits have to do with your child? It's simple. Once you are used to doing these things yourself, you will need to teach them to your child. Since emotions and eating are so intertwined, it will be vital for you to teach your child to manage his or her feelings without using food. The ideas in this chapter will help you do just that. The ways mentioned here of helping your child to break his or her emotional ties to food will provide you with a good beginning. But, as with making changes in family eating habits, be careful not to try to make all of these changes at once. Try one or two small changes as a start, then work toward the others.

The important thing is that you move forward and make progress. Don't worry if a food refusal didn't go as well as you had hoped. Try to treat yourself as you would treat your child when he or she is learning something new. This is not to say that you are childish but only to point out that refusing food and learning to emotionally nourish yourself without food are new practices for many people. And if you are one of these people, it will take time for you to adjust to these new activities. In other words, you wouldn't expect your child to walk for a mile the first time he or she tried, right? More likely, you would expect him or her to start with a shorter distance and work up to the mile. It's the same with your new skills. Since most people are not taught to separate their emotions from food and eating, you are learning a completely new skill.

As a matter of fact, you are learning a skill that is foreign to most Americans as evidenced by the rapidly rising obesity rate. Though it may be difficult, the rewards are many. Both you and your child will learn healthy ways of eating and dealing with your emotions. No longer will food be the focus of holiday events and activities. You will learn to live a healthy lifestyle. But, best of all, your new eating habits will provide you with more energy and enthusiasm for life. It will be easier to move around, and you may even come to like the way your body looks. All of these things are possible for both you and your family. All it takes is some work on your part. In the next chapter, you will learn exactly how to go about making the necessary changes. So roll up your sleeves and get to work. Your child will thank you.

Things to Remember

1. Food and eating are a means of nourishing your body and nothing more.
2. There are many devastating consequences to overeating and being overweight.
3. Advertisers are trying to associate fun and play with high-calorie foods that are unhealthy.

4. Most people spend a lot of time talking about losing weight but do little to make that happen.

5. "Food pushers" will try to coax you into eating things that are unhealthy for you so they don't feel guilty about it.

6. If you feel guilty about setting limits on the types of food your child is eating, nourish yourself in other ways besides eating (hot bath, good book, etc.).

7. Say what you mean. Don't "weaken" and change your mind.

8. Consistency is important when developing new habits.

CHAPTER FIVE

⤞❦⤝

CHANGING THE PATTERNS

SO, THIS IS IT. THE CHAPTER YOU'VE been waiting for—the one that will tell you exactly how to go about helping your child to live a healthier life. Before plunging in, you need to remember that not all of the methods presented here will work for every family. Since people and lifestyles are quite different, you will need to decide what methods will be successful with *your* family. Though this may sound easy, you may face some difficulty in making these determinations. Since, as a member of American society, you have become accustomed to many of the activities that regularly associate food with emotions, you may find yourself resisting all of the methods presented here. This is where your biggest challenge will come—being able to put aside the food denial that is so prevalent in our society in order to determine what is best for you and your family.

The majority of Americans go through life simply maintaining the status quo that they became accustomed to in childhood. This, in part, helps to explain the growing obesity rate among children. Adults learn certain habits and practices from their parents and then pass them on to their children. For instance, passing down certain recipes, holiday-eating traditions, eating habits (such as eating while watching television, only eating in the kitchen, taking food from others' plates, etc.), and taste preferences are all practices that are usually continued from generation to generation without conscious consideration.

What you are being asked to do in this chapter is to become conscious of, and possibly change, habits and practices that were ingrained into your family well before you were even born. This being so, it is easy to see why your resistance to these suggestions might be strong. So what can you do to get past this resistance? First, read each suggestion carefully before going on to the next. If you rush through or skip around this chapter, you may not retain all of the information you need to make an informed decision.

When you do find yourself becoming resistant to one or more of the suggestions presented in this chapter, try to think about where this resistance comes from. If, for example, you read about finding different ways to celebrate holidays rather than baking cookies and you find yourself resisting this, take a second to think about why. What do you associate with baking these cookies? What are you afraid of if you don't bake for the holiday? In your mind, what will happen if there aren't any cookies? What emotions do you associate with this activity? You may want to make a list of the memories you have of baking cookies with your family as a child.

Now, try to figure out if your resistance to taking the advice presented in this chapter is due to a genuine belief that the suggestion mentioned is wrong for your family or rather to a fear of losing the feelings associated with the activity. For example, a child who felt as if the only time he or she had his or her parent's full attention was when they were baking for the holidays may be fearful of losing that parent's love if cookies aren't part of the holiday celebration. Therefore, the resistance here is due to a fear of losing parental love, not a determination that doing without the cookies will in some way harm the family.

Though it may require a change in your thinking, you will need to give each suggestion fair consideration. The best way to do this is to read each suggestion thoroughly and consider whether you experience resistance to it. If you do, wait a few hours or, if possible, think about it overnight before making a final decision. And remember that being uncomfortable about doing something is not a good reason to not do it. Chances are that most of the activities suggested here *will* be uncomfortable, as is the case with most life changes. Think again about your child learning a new skill. Do you think he or she felt comfortable at first? Of course not. Whether it's learning to horseback ride, play basketball, or anything else, it took some time for him or her to feel comfortable, just as it will for you when implementing these suggestions.

If this chapter seems overwhelming to you, there is a good reason. In an attempt to present as many alternatives as possible, a great deal of information has been packed into the following pages. Since there are so many different types of people and families, it is certain that no one method will work for everyone. What follows is an attempt to try and offer a large number of tips and suggestions in the hope that most families will be able to use at least one. I hope, however, that many more will appeal to you. It bears repeating that I encourage you to pick and choose what works for you and your family. Under no circumstances should you try to do everything outlined in this chapter. Try one or two approaches and see how they work in your family.

Also don't be afraid to abandon the ones that don't work for you and/or your family. What's written here may read well on paper but be difficult or impractical when you try to implement it in your life. That's perfectly acceptable. Simply move on to another suggestion then determine whether or not that one works for you and your child. Remember that what *you* think will work for your child may be very different from what he or she thinks; therefore, it will be necessary for you to try a variety of the ideas mentioned here.

Now, it's time to begin. Be consistent. If you're like most parents, the last thing you want to do at the end of the day is put together an elaborate meal. This is exactly the sort of thing that the major fast-food restaurants count on. Think of the slogan "You deserve a break today." While this may be true, if you're going to improve your child's health, you will need to find a healthier means of creating fast food. One of the best methods of doing this starts with a trip to your local supermarket. Today, many supermarkets include hot foods to go. Among these offerings are roasted chicken and turkey. Either is a good alternative to greasy hamburgers.

In the produce aisle, you can now find precut fruit and vegetables that can be incorporated into a meal with little effort. For instance, a stir-fry package of vegetables often includes broccoli, cauliflower, snow peas, and carrots. Combine this in a skillet with a little soy sauce and you have a vegetable that may even appeal to your children. If your child likes spicy foods, then you may try adding red pepper, hot sauce, or ginger, too. In the produce aisle, you will also find peeled and cubed potatoes. These potatoes can be quickly boiled to provide a healthy substitute for high-calorie french-fries. Even if your child won't eat them without a little butter, this alternative is still better than the fried version. Since the potatoes are cut into small cubes, boiling them won't take long—or you may want to use the microwave to speed things up even more.

If these foods don't appeal to you, try the salad bar. Salad bars in grocery stores are filled with a wide variety of fresh vegetables. Be careful, however, not to pour on high-fat and high-calorie dressing. This will only counteract what you are trying to accomplish. At the deli counter, premade sandwiches or even sliced lunchmeat can be purchased. Again, be careful about the dressing. Many stores make it a practice to smother oil and vinegar all over these sandwiches. Since oil has only a slight taste, you can usually skip it without sacrificing flavor. Mayonnaise is very high in fat, but mustard and ketchup are not unhealthy choices. Or you can always purchase your own meat and enlist the help of your child to make sandwiches for dinner.

If your child is accustomed to having dessert after a meal, it could cause resentment if you simply stopped serving it. A better alternative is to include healthy desserts. Many supermarkets have pre- or partially cut fruit that can be substituted for these high-calorie dessert items. Depending on the season, you may find watermelon, cantaloupe, honeydew, pineapples, or even strawberries. If precut fruit is not available in your supermarket, consider using fruit "precut" by nature, such as grapes, cherries, bananas, etc. Though it may take a few tries for your child to get used to some of these fruits, if you are patient and consistent, it will happen.

Another immediate action that you can take to improve your child's health is to build on those healthy foods that he or she already likes. If your child does like fruit, be sure to have it in the house regularly. Though this may seem like common sense, it's easy to forget. If you're worried that your child won't eat the fruit before it goes bad, buy canned fruit in its own juice. With today's canning methods, this type of fruit is sometimes healthier than what you find in the produce aisle.

Being sure that your child has between three and five structured meals is also vital to helping your child develop healthier eating habits. Developing set meal times will go a long way toward eliminating emotional eating. It's not just common sense; one study published in a national magazine devoted to health issues showed that kids who had dinner with their parents ate lower-fat foods and more fruits and veggies. In contrast, overweight children reported eating at least half of their meals in front of the television. Structured mealtimes with beginnings and endings implicitly discourage prolonged "grazing" throughout the day. This will help your child to develop boundaries around eating rather than viewing it as a recreational activity.

In line with this, practice portion control. The size of the portion presented to eaters helps determine the amount they consume. According to a study by a Pennsylvania State nutritionist, lean young men, known to regulate food intake well, were influenced by the size of the portions presented to them to eat more food. When served 16 ounces, they ate 10, but when given a 25-ounce "jumbo lunch," they ate 15 ounces, 50 percent more than what had satisfied them previously. So much for "regulating food intake well."

Imagine this scenario with an already overweight child. Portion control, therefore, becomes vital in your efforts to help your child lose weight.

Rather than "telling" your child to limit his or her portion, instead make only enough food for one meal. Though it may be more convenient to cook meals in advance, when beginning this program, you may need to follow the suggested serving sizes listed on food packages. Cook and serve enough for the current meal. It may take some practice to determine the correct amounts. Most of what is portioned out at restaurants is much greater than nutritionally acceptable amounts of food. This being so, determining proper portions may take practice but it will be worth it when considering your child's health.

Watching television while eating should be avoided. While this may seem to be common practice in America, think about the message being sent to your child. Watching television is a recreational activity that's meant to be fun. By allowing children to eat in front of the television, you are associating eating with this fun activity, very similar to the way movie theaters have us trained to equate eating popcorn with watching feature films. Dinnertime should be simply the period during the day when you take time out to nourish your body. It should not be equated with watching television, playing games on the computer, or any other play activity.

In addition to this, studies have shown that people tend to eat more while watching television. As author Marie Winn points out in her book, *The Plug-In Drug*, "The explanation of why television viewing might lead to obesity seems obvious: 1. If you're watching, you're not doing something more active and 2. While you're watching you're likely to be snacking." To add to this, Winn points to a Memphis State University study that found that children watching television had metabolic rates similar to that of sleeping, while the levels of those "sitting there doing nothing," were significantly higher. "The effect was even greater for overweight children. Since the metabolic rate measures the number of calories a person uses up over time, this finding demonstrates that it's not merely a matter of TV watching displacing some form of exercise that encourages obesity. By reducing the metabolic rate, the act of TV watching itself makes kids more likely to be fat." This reason alone should be enough to turn off the television.

Taking this a step further, you may want to consider taking the television set out of your child's room if there is one present—that's one way to limit the number of food ads your child sees. According to a study by the Kaiser Family Foundation, "Today, 8–18 year-olds devote an average of 7 hours and 38 minutes (7:38) to using entertainment media across a typical day (more than 53 hours a week). And because they spend so much of that time 'media multitasking' (using more than one medium at a time), they actually manage to pack a total of 10 hours and 45 minutes (10:45) worth of media content into those 7½ hours. "

Add to this the fact that children have access to many different types of media and you can see how serious the problem is. As the Kaiser study points out, "The amount of time spent with media increased by 1 hour and 17 minutes a day over the past five years, from 6:21 in 2004 to 7:38 today. And because of media multitasking, the total amount of media content consumed during that period has increased from 8:33 in 2004 to 10:45 today."

Furthermore, according to a study by the Rudd Center, "Advertising for the least nutritious categories of food including fast food; cereal; carbonated beverages; and juice, fruit drinks, and sports drinks declined in 2011, but youth exposure to candy advertising from 2009 to 2011 increased by 55 to 70 percent."

While the previous suggestions concentrate more on the physical aspects of eating, the following ones will address the emotional aspects often associated with food. To begin, it is vital that you don't use food as means of controlling your child's actions. It has become common practice to effectively bribe children for good behavior. Here a few examples of this:

"If you clean your room, we'll go for ice cream."

"If you're good during the ride home, I'll buy you a candy bar."

"If you eat your vegetables, you'll get dessert."

"When you finish your homework, you can have a cookie."

Though most of these statements seem to be an ordinary part of American life, think for a second about the ramifications of putting greater importance on certain types of foods than on others. Not only does it give your child the message that dessert items are more desirable, it associates feelings of accomplishment and parental approval with food and eating. In other words, at the same time you are trying to teach your children positive behaviors, you are also teaching them to associate eating high-calorie foods with accomplishment. Using food as a means of rewarding children sets up a pattern that will be carried into adulthood and that can be lifelong. Remember the example at the beginning of this book about a child being presented with a lollipop after a visit to the dentist? The examples presented here operate on the same idea—using food as a reward.

The danger here is that as a child grows older, he or she will come to not only expect rewards for good behavior but to expect high-calorie foods, thus setting up unhealthy patterns that will be passed down to his or her own children. Rather than offering food as a reward, try to think of a healthy alternative. Does your child like to climb trees? Read? Play catch? Collect stuffed animals? Write? Draw? Whatever it is, if you do find it necessary to reward your child, using food is not the best way. If you have been regularly rewarding your child with food, then slowly begin to introduce the alternatives above, if they are things he or she enjoys. Rather than using food every time, for example, try alternating between food and something else. Then move to every third or fourth time until finally you have replaced food rewards entirely.

Expanding on this, attempts to control your child's food intake will only result in frustration for you both. If you overtly begin to try and limit your child's food intake, you are once again causing your child to associate feelings with food. Think about your own childhood. If your parents told you not to do something, what was the first thing you wanted to do? Exactly what they told you not to, right? Well, it works the same with food. The more you protest your child's food choices, the more appealing they become to him or her. This will eventually cause your child to associate feelings of freedom and adulthood with food and eating, once again setting up unhealthy lifelong eating patterns.

Rather than struggle with your child over his or her food choices, do what you can to set an example. Explain how important healthy eating is for a healthy body and do not make high-calorie food available in your house. At dinnertime, simply put several healthy choices on the table and let your child decide what he or she will eat. Either way, if you only offer healthy choices, your child will be forced to choose something nutritious. By allowing your child to make choices, you are giving him or her freedom within certain parameters.

Should your child refuse to eat anything, simply state that this is what you have made for dinner and if he or she chooses not to eat any of it, no other alternatives will be offered. Resist the temptation to offer alternatives. Instead, if your child chooses to abstain from eating, simply allow him or her to be excused from the table. Do not punish him or her and do not continuously ask whether or not he or she is hungry. Simply allow your child the freedom not to eat what is presented at dinnertime. If it is your custom to offer your child a snack before bedtime, then do so as you normally would. Again, only offer healthy choices and let your child decide. Should he or she ask to eat a bedtime snack after dinner, make two or three acceptable suggestions then let your child decide.

Though you may experience feelings of guilt, try to hang tough. Your child will eat something soon enough. He or she will not starve to death. Instead, his or her biological needs will become too strong to be ignored. You are not a bad parent if your child chooses not to eat the food you have presented. Your love for your child is not measured by how much or how little he or she eats. Quite the opposite, by teaching your child to eat healthy, you are setting up lifelong patterns that will serve your child well throughout his or her life. Though it's not easy, it is necessary.

Another important method of separating emotions from food is to educate your child about the advertising industry. If you and your child watch television together, initiate a conversation about advertisers and their motives. Use a commercial for food to let your child know that eating certain foods does not make life better or more fun in the way that it is portrayed on television. In many schools across the country, children are taught media evaluation skills. These skills will go a long way in helping your child take the emotional aspects out of eating. If your child's curriculum does not include media evaluation or if you'd like to reinforce what he or she is learning in school, begin by pointing out that the sole purpose of advertisements, no matter how funny or cute they may be is to sell products. Food advertisements certainly do not point out the negative consequences of overconsuming unhealthy foods.

How often is your child exposed to the consequences of eating too much unhealthy food? Probably not very often, if at all. To do so would cause food manufacturers to lose money. Think for a second: if food manufacturers had to include warning labels in the same manner that cigarette companies are forced to, they might read something like this: "Overeating this product may cause obesity resulting in heart disease, high blood pressure, and elevated cholesterol levels." Sounds ridiculous, doesn't it?

Yet, consider the fact that each day millions of already overweight people regularly eat foods high in calories despite the fact that the Framingham Heart Study, a landmark study begun in Massachusetts in 1948, found solid evidence of a link between heart failure and excessive weight, citing a risk of heart failure that is 34 percent higher among overweight individuals and 104 percent higher for obese people.

Since the study was first done, it has been repeated throughout the years, consistently proving that high blood pressure, heart disease, and high cholesterol can be controlled by lifestyle changes. To date, over one thousand published medical papers are related to the original study. Now, add to this the fact that according to many experts, more than 800 people die each day as a result of obesity, and that number is growing.

Even with knowledge about the dangers of overeating, Americans continue to overeat. Perhaps this is due in part out of ignorance; but even more so, it may be attributed to a lack of realistic media portrayals regarding food and eating. Open any women's magazine and you will find a very thin woman "bragging" about eating high-calorie items. Perhaps *she* does; but her experiences are shaped by her unique metabolism and lifestyle, yet readers will carry away the message that there is something wrong with *them* if they eat as much as she does and are overweight. And, of course, magazine features may exaggerate or report what the interviewee says unquestioningly. Really, how many high-calorie foods can this woman possibly eat and still maintain her shape? The answer is obviously very few. As an adult you may be aware of this media tendency to distort reality, but what about similar content in children's magazines or on television? Can you be certain that children are as aware of the duplicity in these publications?

The point here is that you should take every possible opportunity to communicate with your child about the advertisements and features to which he or she is regularly exposed. You may start by asking him or her what sort of feelings the commercial being viewed brings up and if this is consistent with the actual product being advertised. For example, if you are watching a chocolate commercial where children are participating in physical activity, ask your child how he or she feels about the commercial. You may point out that the children are doing something very physical that they wouldn't be able to do as easily if they ate too much of the chocolate. Explain to your child that being overweight makes it difficult to move around and results in feelings of lethargy rather than energy. It may be helpful to try and make a game out of identifying the feelings advertisers are attempting to portray and contrast them with those that actually result from using the products advertised. If you are patient and persistent, your child will eventually get the message even if he or she is unwilling to admit it to you.

It's important to remember, when doing this or any of the activities outlined here, that your child may not be receptive to your efforts. That's okay. Your child has the right to resist what he or she may see as an attack on your family's lifestyle. Simply make an attempt then wait a few days and try again. If, after three tries, he or she is still as resistant as in the beginning, then move onto something else. Remember, you are not trying to do every activity in this book perfectly. This is impossible. It will take time and effort on your part to bring about permanent changes in your child's eating habits. You are attempting to change years of established habits; therefore, you need to be patient and understanding when it is difficult for your child. Allow him or her the opportunity to refuse to participate in one or more of the activities you suggest but be open to the future possibilities.

In line with this, it's also worth pointing out that there are some events beyond your control. While you are able to control the types of food that are brought into your house, you cannot control what your child does at a friend's house or at other outside activities. If, for example, it has been your child's custom to stop at a burger joint with a friend twice a week, you may not want to put a stop to this abruptly. Instead, you may try to offer a healthier alternative; but if your child resists, let it go for now. Concentrate on making changes in your home. The goal isn't to be perfect; it is to improve your child's eating habits. Since children are constantly offered candy and other high-calorie items at parties and school events as a routine practice, you will not be able to control every single item that goes into your child's mouth. Nor should you try.

Excluding your child from parties or festive events will only cause resentment on your child's part. Unfortunately, most child-centered events include high-calorie sweets. To prohibit your child from attending may cause ridicule from other children. The fact is that eating these items once in a while will not hurt your child. Your concentration should be on the day-to-day events that you do have a say in. Once again, if high-calorie dessert items are not in your house, it will be much more difficult for your child to eat them. That is your arena. To try and change society all at once would not only be foolish but frustrating as well.

Rather than trying to change everyone and everything at once, your best bet is to take small steps. A lot of major changes at once will cause your child to feel unsafe and insecure, which may result in him or her seeking more food to help deal with these feelings. You are not trying to change your child's entire life. You are only making one or two small changes at a time to help your child eat healthier. You cannot undo a lifetime of conditioning in a week and it would be dangerous to try. Be systematic and consistent. These are the two most important aspects of making any change. Once you begin, be sure to follow through. Do not make changes for a few days or weeks then go back to doing things the way you always have. Again, this will cause confusion and even resentment from your child.

In the beginning, although you may encounter a great deal of resistance from your child when you begin to make these changes, if you are consistent, your child will eventually come around. Do not engage in debates or power struggles with your child. Simply state that you are trying to make changes in your lifestyle and you are no longer comfortable with having high-calorie dessert items in your house. Your child may whine and complain about this. That's to be expected. He or she is trying to change your mind. The best weapon you have in your fight for your child's health is your persistence. Do not yell at or fight with your child. Simply state that this is the way it will be from now on and stick to it. Your child will eventually get used to this and may even come to appreciate your efforts.

Even when it seems difficult to continue with your new way of life, you must not give up. If you stop doing what you've begun, your child will get the message that you aren't serious about eating healthy and he or she will use this as a reason to overeat. Your child will view healthy eating as a passing fad rather than a way of life. Inconsistency will promote the diet mentality that so many Americans are familiar with. A diet is something that has a beginning and an end. A new way of life, however, should be a consistent undertaking. If you give up, you are ultimately teaching your child to do the same.

Another important method of helping your child to attain healthy eating patterns is to encourage your child to develop interests outside of food and eating. Though this may seem like a very basic activity, think about it for a second. If your child is involved in a hobby, then he or she is not eating. To begin, think about the kinds of things that you enjoyed as a child. Consider sharing one or two of these with your child (or perhaps you can share a hobby you currently enjoy, if it is suitable). If putting together models was something you enjoyed, why not work on one with your child? Or if you quilting is your passion, introduce your child to this. Be sure to ask your child if he or she is interested in trying your hobby. If not, do not apply pressure. Rather, ask your child what sort of thing he or she is interested in then encourage this.

For many overweight children, eating becomes a hobby. Though this may not be as blatant as it is described here, eating is involved in many children's interests. Going to the movies generally involves eating popcorn or candy. Watching television is many times paired with eating snacks. A day at the beach usually includes ice cream. Many after-school activities involve snacking on cookies and candy, while camping is paired with toasting marshmallows. There are many other examples of activities that are generally associated with eating, but the point here remains the same—encourage your child to find interests that do not involve food. Some of these may include horseback riding, playing softball, ice skating, skiing, rollerblading, playing football, dancing, karate, swimming, yoga, or basketball. Be sure to encourage, not pressure, your child. If he or she isn't interested in a certain activity, move on to another one.

You may also want to consider volunteer work. If, for example, your child is interested in animals, then perhaps a few hours a week at a local animal shelter would be a positive experience. Or if your child loves horses or a particular dog breed, there are many horse rescue and other animal rescue organizations that need help. This will not only be a good way to get your child acquainted with the benefits of volunteering, it will also allow him or her to meet other people interested in the same things he or she is.

Another way to help your child develop healthy eating habits is to educate him or her about the benefits of eating healthy foods. If your child is younger, you can make a game out of memorizing the names of certain fruits and vegetables. If your child is a little older, you may present him or her with the challenge of discovering what vitamins are present in certain foods and how they serve to nourish the human body.

If you are dealing with a teenager, you may point to interesting articles about nutrition; or if you're worried about encountering resistance, simply leave the articles in an area where your child is likely to see them, perhaps on the table, in the bathroom, or even in the family room. With a little practice, you will find what works for your child. And no matter what the activity, remember that the point of it is to educate your child about the benefits of healthy eating. A little knowledge can go a long way in changing destructive eating habits.

Similarly, you may also want to educate your child about the consequences of obesity. With a little research at your local library or a quick trip online, you can easily find information about the dangers of being overweight. Whatever you decide, it is vital that your child realizes that there are consequences to being overweight.

As you have already read, advertisers spend large amounts of money to convince children that eating their products is fun. These efforts by advertisers make it difficult for most children to realize that there are long-term physical consequences to being overweight. Though your child may be skeptical about the information you present, it is necessary to make him or her aware of these consequences. Again, be sure not to overwhelm your child with volumes. Rather choose one or two articles or programs that you think your child will find helpful. After presenting the information to your child, let him or her initiate any conversation about the material. Your part in this matter is to simply introduce your child to the information then simply let your child do what he or she will with it.

The most important method of helping your child to "de-emotionalize" food is to educate him or her about how to express feelings in a constructive manner. In general, most people are not educated about expressing feelings; rather, as a society, we are taught to hide our feelings behind polite smiles. So, if you've never been taught how to express your feelings in a healthy way, where do you begin? Well, depending on the level of awareness you have, it may be necessary to seek professional help. If you already have some knowledge, then you can use it to benefit your child.

To begin, model for your child a way to express his or her feelings by using *I statements* to express your own feelings. This involves saying "I feel _____ when you _____." Notice that the first word in the sentence is "I." The most important part of expressing feelings is to take ownership of them. Using the word "I" does this. Rather than saying "You make me angry," by beginning the sentence with the word "I," the speaker takes ownership of his or her feelings, which in turn causes the speaker to take responsibility for them.

It may also be necessary for you to educate your child about the difference between feelings and judgments. Feelings, for example, can usually be broken down with four basic words—sad, mad, glad, and afraid. Judgments, however, evaluate those feelings. For instance, saying, "I feel rejected," does not describe a feeling but is rather an evaluation. Rejection is subjective, dependent on each person's interpretation of a certain standard. Generally, the feeling behind rejection is sadness, fear, or even anger. "Rejection" is not an expression of feelings; it is a characterization of the actions of another in relation to oneself.

Another valuable tool in encouraging your child to express his or her feelings is writing. In the same way that you used writing in Chapter Two to list your family's eating habits, your child can use writing to express feelings. If your child is sad or angry, for example, suggest that he or she write about the experience. Or taking it a step further, you may encourage your child to keep a journal. Whatever method you suggest, be certain that you do not try to read what your child has written unless he or she asks you to. The kind of writing that is necessary for your child to express his or her feelings is personal and should be kept private unless the person doing the writing requests otherwise. Your child needs to feel as if he or she has a safe place to express feelings without fear of the consequences. By supporting your child in this, you will be offering a valuable lesson about separating feelings from food.

If your child complains that he or she has nothing to write about, you may try to make a few suggestions or perhaps even keep a journal yourself and share your experience with your child. First, you may suggest that your child make a list of ten things that he or she likes to do. If your child chooses to share this list with you, then you can use it to encourage promising hobbies or activities. Another writing exercise that may help your child learn to express his or her feelings is to write about the happiest, saddest, most exciting, etc. event. This will help your child to identify feelings and relate them to experiences. Following is a list of suggested writing prompts for your child. But, again, remember not to force anything, and don't present all of them at once.

- What makes you feel better when you are sad?
- Write a story about a child who is very happy. Why is he or she happy?
- What is the safest place you know? What makes it so safe?
- Make a list of the five most precious things in your life.
- Name the three qualities about yourself that you like the most.
- Write about your favorite outfit. How do you feel when you wear it?
- If you could change one thing about yourself, what would it be? Why?
- If a fairy gave you three wishes, what would they be?
- Write about your favorite book or movie. What do you like about it?
- What is your favorite color? What does it make you think about?

- If you could live in a different time period, which one would you choose? Why?
- Write about a time when you accomplished something you were proud of.
- If you were an athlete, what sport would you participate in? Why?

While some of these writing exercises may need to be adjusted for the age of your child, the goal here is for your child to become more self-aware. The more your child knows about him- or herself, the better chance there is of separating emotions from food. If your child is especially young and unable to write yet, you may be able to present these activities as a game. Cut out pictures from magazines and ask your child to arrange the objects in order of preference. What is most appealing and why? You can do this with colors, clothes, music, animated characters, flowers, sports equipment, book covers, etc. Just about anything will work—but do not use anything associated with food.

If your child decides to share the writings with you, do not comment either negatively or positively. Simply listen without judgment. While you may ask questions about something you don't understand, do not try to change your child's mind about anything. If, for example, food or eating is mentioned on any of the lists, simply listen. Trying to change your child's mind about anything, especially food, will set up a power struggle, causing your child to feel attacked and therefore need to defend his or her choices. By simply offering a sympathetic ear, you will become your child's ally rather than his or her adversary.

If the writing is particularly upsetting to you, it's important that you consider why before making any comment to your child. Since this may take some time, the best thing you can do is to simply ask a neutral question or share a similar experience of your own. If you are at a complete loss as to what to say, simply ask your child how he or she felt while writing. Remember that no matter what your child has written, they are just words on paper; and these words are simply a reflection of your child's feelings on any given day. This situation is not permanent. Feelings are constantly changing. Your child's are no exception to this.

On the other hand, if your child expressed feelings that repeatedly mention suicidal thoughts or depression, then you need to contact an expert immediately. Such statements should not be taken lightly.

Should you find something upsetting in your child's writing, you will need to look at it further. To begin, think about why what your child wrote is upsetting you. Are you being overly sensitive or is something genuinely upsetting in the writing? Is your child simply expressing feelings that you don't like or are you taking these feelings as a criticism of your parenting skills? Either way, you need to remind yourself that whatever your child's feelings are, it is not your responsibility to fix or change them. Though it may be difficult for you to hear that your child is unhappy about something in life, it's best to give him or her some time to try and work it out without interfering. By doing this, you will provide your child with much-needed problem-solving skills.

You may even question your child about what can be done to make the situation better. Beware, though. Your child may try to put responsibility on you for making the situation better. To do so would be a mistake on your part. Instead, ask your child what *he or she* can do to improve the situation. Sometimes this will simply be a matter of finding alternative behaviors or activities. Whatever it is, let your child come up with the solution and make sure that it doesn't involve food or eating. If your child does try to suggest eating something to make things better, simply ask if that's the best way the situation can be handled. You may offer one or two suggestions if your child is unable to think of alternatives but leave it up to your child to decide the course of action to be taken.

If writing isn't something your child enjoys, then think about crafts or even exercises that the whole family can do. Following is a list of suggestions. Again, only choose the ones that feel right for you and your family.

Craft Exercises
- Draw a picture of a place where you feel safe.
- Cut pictures out of a magazine and make a collage of things you love.
- Draw a picture of something that makes you feel special.
- Trace your hands on a piece of paper then make a list of things you love to do with your hands that make you happy.
- Draw a picture of yourself ten years from now.
- Using photos, magazines, and newspapers, create a "happy page."
- Draw a picture of what sadness looks like.
- Draw a picture of what happiness looks like.
- Make a picture of a star and write your name in the middle. Color it in.
- Draw a picture of an award you would like to earn.

Family Exercises

- For one week, each member of the family takes three minutes to talk about his or her feelings during the day.

- Each family member talks about what makes him or her happy then what makes him or her sad.

- Cut out pictures from magazines that describe the four basic feelings—sad, mad, glad, scared—then ask each member of the family to talk about a time when he or she felt each of these. Do not interrupt each other.

- While at a park or the beach, each member of the family collects (or points to) three things that he or she likes and talks about why he or she likes these things.

- Each member of the family draws a picture or uses family or magazine photos to create a picture of a place that makes him or her feel safe.

- Over the course of a week, each family member chooses one person, either living or deceased, whom he or she admires, finds out information about this person's life, then shares this with other family members.

- Taking turns, each person talks about three special things about the other family members, being careful to only mention positive traits.

- During the week, each family member must make a list describing at least one special thing that other family members have done for him or her over the past seven days then discuss it together.

- Each member of the family writes a letter to a person he or she admires. After the letters are written, everyone takes turns reading them.

- After playing a game (Scrabble, Monopoly, etc.), each member of the family talks about how he or she felt, both while participating and the results.

- Organize a craft night. Once a week each family member introduces a craft or activity that he or she likes. Everyone participates then talks about how it went.

Your most important weapon in the war on childhood obesity is your ability to "de-emotionalize" food. Emotions include both so-called positive and negative feelings. Try to keep emotions separate from food choices. This can mean that if your child reaches for a high-calorie dessert item while you are both at a party, do not make a scene or try to change the choice. Don't let your emotions dictate your reaction although you may be disappointed or concerned. Simply allow your child to make the food choices. In the same way that you allow this in your home when the choices are healthy, you must be consistent—even if there is high-calorie food involved. Again, if you tell your child not to eat something, especially if you do so with emotion, that item will become even more attractive and possibly be used in the future as a display of freedom or rebellion.

By taking the emotions out of the food battle, you are allowing your child the chance to make food decisions based on taste. Though this may seem risky, realize that your number one priority is to break the association your child has between food and emotions. In order to accomplish this, you will need to allow your child the opportunity to make choices on a regular basis. In your home, those choices are limited among healthy foods. Outside the home, however, the choices may not be between items that are as healthy, but it's vital that you still allow your child to choose.

Another way of helping your child to take the emotions out of food is to develop new habits that don't revolve around food. In the same way that you encouraged your child to develop his or her own interests apart from food, it will be necessary to develop healthy family habits as well. If it has become your custom to take your child to the fast-food playland on weekends, why not try an outdoor playground or public park? Or maybe an indoor roller rink or miniature golf course? If you and your child regularly have ice cream together after school, how about trying a walk or a game of catch instead? More suggestions on how to incorporate exercise will be included in the next chapter. For now, just try to be aware of the habits you have developed as a family and try to make changes where you can.

Before concluding this chapter, it is necessary to discuss the resistance you may face within yourself. *The Plug-In Drug* lists ten reasons parents can't control TV. Winn's reasons parents can't control television viewing are translated below as related to healthy eating. (Where necessary, the word "eating" has been substituted for viewing.)

Ten Reasons Parents Can't Control Overeating

1. Fear of Saying "No"

Winn points out that many parents are simply afraid to deny their children anything. Relating this to food, there can be some fear involved in denying children something as basic as food. Since many of our parents and grandparents grew up in a time when food was scarce, even rationed, saying no to your child's food requests may seem tyrannical, even cruel. Yet, saying no or limiting your child's food choices is the healthiest thing you can do for your child.

For some, saying no may mean that your child will become angry with you, which brings with it a fear that your child won't love you anymore. While this may be one of your fears, it's important to realize that to refrain from saying no because you are afraid of losing your child's love is selfish, as you are putting your concerns before the welfare of your child. In other words, saying no is not fun, but it is necessary. If this is particularly troublesome or difficult for you, you may want to seek outside support to help you deal with this. Enlist the help of a friend or perhaps a counselor. No matter what you do, it is important that you learn to say no when your child asks you to bring unhealthy food into the house.

2. The Parents' Own Eating Habits

As Winn indicates, "Frequently, parents' own viewing habits nullify their attempts to reduce their children's dependence on television. Parents who themselves have come to depend on television for amusement, relaxation, or escape find it hard to set limits on their children's viewing." Think about this as it relates to food. If you want your child to eat healthy, you will need to eat healthy as well. Having only healthy food in the house will mean that you will not have ready access to high-calorie junk food. It may also mean that you will have to put some extra work into preparing meals or grocery shopping.

As you read earlier, your child's healthy eating habits begin with you. If you are not ready to make changes in your own diet, then you are certainly not prepared to help your child. Though you will not have to give up every last bit of junk food, it will be necessary to make certain changes in your own eating patterns.

3. Will My Child Be a Social Outcast?

Winn states that parents' fear about their child being an outcast is "one of the strongest deterrents to effective television control in American families." Think about this as it relates to food. Were you afraid for your child's welfare when it was suggested that you make changes in his or her activities? Do all or most of the people you know take their child to fast-food restaurants? Were you afraid that your child would lose friends if you eliminated this activity?

While this may seem to be a valid fear, think about the words of one father who limits his children to two hours of television a week. "I used to say to my kids, 'Your friends are going to like you because of the way you behave—whether you're generous or friendly or fun to be with —and not because you've watched the same TV shows they watch. It's who you are that matters.'" This is also true of food and eating. Though your child may eventually find new friends who share the new interests he or she has developed, the way your child eats should not deter those friends who truly care about your child.

4. Ambivalence

"Parents' difficulties are compounded by a lack of certainty about what role they wish television to play in their family life and a basic ambivalence about television," according to Winn.

Relating this to food, many parents may feel conflicted about not baking with their children for holidays or not having popcorn at the movies. This results in feelings of ambivalence that tend to confuse children with mixed messages. For instance, many parents waver on their commitment to healthy eating behaviors while expecting that their child will automatically eat healthy.

5. Lack of Conviction

Winn declares that when trying to control children's television viewing, many parents find it to be "too much of a hassle," or "not worth the agony." This may be the case with healthy eating as well. Any parent will surely admit that it is much easier to give in to a child rather than standing your ground. Even those who are able to stand firm most times, yet give in occasionally, are sending mixed messages about healthy eating to their children. As Winn notes, "If parents want to control their children's television watching, they have to make it clear that it's as important as not playing with sharp knives or running into a busy street."

It's the same with healthy eating. If you are to get your message across, it must be a firm, strong message that's consistent at all times.

6. Lack of Confidence

Winn points to the "diminishing authority of the family" as being a reason that parents are anxious about regulating children's habits. She quotes a mother of three to illustrate her point. "What's wrong with me is that I don't know what's right and what's wrong and neither do my children. Now, my mother, to this day, believes in right and wrong, and she believes she knows what's right and what's wrong. But I absolutely don't. Outside of a very few moral issues, I don't know what's right or wrong about a lot of things . . . ."

This woman's frustration could most likely be doubled when discussing nutritional information. As we've already discussed, the media are filled with contradictory "facts" about healthy eating, so confusion is only natural. Yet, letting this confusion get in the way of your confidence when helping your child to eat healthy, could cause harm to your child's health.

Again, common sense should be the guide here when trying to determine a healthy eating plan for your child. Find someone you trust. Your child's doctor is a good start. Research what's out there but be wary of any plan that excludes what you already know to be healthy—vegetables, fruits, etc. Once you have decided on a general eating plan, follow whatever guidelines you establish and stick with them. This will help you to gain confidence in your choices.

7. Parental Lack of Agreement

Consider Winn's example of one father who had trouble saying no to his five-year-old's television watching. "I didn't really think television was so bad; I didn't think it was worth the struggle since he wanted to watch so badly. But now the television stays off even if he throws a fit. An hour a day, that's the rule and we stick to it. Once it was established, Peter caught on quickly. But when my wife and I were not completely in agreement about television, he saw right away that this was a great opportunity to bug us, to drive a wedge between us."

Think about this where healthy eating is concerned. How many times have you or your partner said no to something only to have the other turn around and offer it to the child? Though it may be difficult, you and your child's other parent must find a way to present a united front about eating healthy.

8. A Misguided Pursuit of Democracy

Winn notes that some parents believe being strict is undemocratic. "They fear that by laying down the law about television—or indeed, about anything else—they will cause their children to grow up overly rebellious or overly docile. As a result they find that their natural authority as parents and adults is undermined and their ability to control television at home is weakened."

When relating this to food, you can see the danger involved if parents refuse to take a strong stance on healthy eating. One of the most self-defeating things you can do when trying to change your child's eating habits is to give him or her mixed messages about eating. If for instance, you tell your child not to eat candy, then bring home a pack of candy bars from the grocery store, your child will become confused and maybe try to change your mind. Though our country is democratic, healthy eating among children should not be. While your child has the right to make choices within the parameters you set, no child should be given free reign to eat anything and everything.

This may be difficult and cause you to feel guilty but it is important not to give in. "I know it sounds weak, but I just hate to be the one to be constantly disappointing people, regulating them, stopping them from doing something they enjoy. I don't like to be the heavy in the family. I'd rather we were all on equal footing . . .." This mother's words exemplify the concept of misguided democracy. The truth, however, is that being a parent means setting some difficult rules that may make you feel guilty and temporarily place you squarely in the path of your child's anger. You will need to learn how to manage your own feelings. Seek support from other parents or professionals; but whatever happens, don't give in to letting your child eat foods that you know are unhealthy. In the same way that you wouldn't let your child play with a loaded gun, you need to be equally strict in setting boundaries around food.

9. Devaluation of Parents' Rights

Winn points out that devaluation of parents' rights leads to "acceptance of a child-centered philosophy of raising children" that causes parents to see "life exclusively from [their] children's point of view." Winn uses a "harried young mother['s]" words to illustrate her point. "When my kids are being awful and rude while I'm talking on the phone, instead of disciplining them, there's a part of me that says, 'Yes, I'm on the phone too long.'" According to Winn, this mother has "lost her perspective" by putting the child's desires above her own.

Relating this to food, you can see how dangerous looking at eating from your child's point of view could be. Your child is exactly that—a child. Putting his or her health first is not a consideration for most children. This is where your role as parent comes into the picture. In order for your child to develop healthy eating patterns, it will be necessary for you to reclaim your parental rights and set tough limits that may cause your child to be temporarily unhappy. Again, you will need to learn to live with your feelings about setting firm boundaries for your child. Even the most child-centered parent would have to agree that a parent's role involves taking responsibility for a child's health and safety until he or she is old enough to do it him- or herself.

10. Sleep Deprivation

Winn points out that many parents use television as a babysitter to gain more sleep time. This may also be the case with food. Think about how many times you may have suggested that your child eat something while you sleep in on the weekend. Do you regularly entertain your children with food while you rest in the afternoon? Either way, as Winn notes, ". . . for a family dominated by television, in the long run it may be worth losing a bit of sleep to gain control of that powerful medium." The same holds true for food.

Now that you have read the ten reasons that it is difficult for parents to control their children's overeating, you may want to take another few minutes to read them again. Though they were originally designed for television viewing, these reasons translate well when discussing overeating. For instance, how many times have you been resistant to saying no to your child where food is concerned? As you already know, many parents use food to nurture their children. With this association being in place, it is not difficult to see how denying your children food may be seen as similar to withholding affection from them.

It is important for you to realize that food and affection are only related in advertising—not in real life. As a generation that grew up with the idea that you can "bake someone happy," this may be a difficult concept to grasp, but it is the truth. Food is simply a way to nourish your body. You cannot make someone love you by feeding them. Quite the opposite, your child will benefit more from your loving firmness than he or she could ever from overeating.

By following the suggestions in this chapter, you will not only be taking steps to improve your child's health, but you will begin breaking decades of dangerous patterns that have become firmly established in American society. While food manufacturers have spent billions of dollars to convince you that food is fun, that it demonstrates affection and love and can add excitement to everyday life, you do not need to spend one single cent to realize how very wrong these ideas are. What is being asked of you instead, is to be firm, committed, and consistent when dealing with your child's eating habits. Surely, you can handle that. Now, read on and find out how to make exercise a part of your family routine. And, remember, your child is worth all of the effort you are putting into the practices outlined in this book.

Things to Remember

There are many suggestions in this chapter. Not all of them will work for every family, nor should you try to do every one mentioned.

1. Be consistent when trying a new activity. It's best to start slowly.
2. Don't use food to control your child's actions.
3. Do not engage in power struggles over food with your child.
4. Never give up even when it seems hard. Given time, this will work.

5. Help your child to express his or her feelings by using some of the exercises mentioned in this chapter.

6. Journaling is a helpful way to help children understand themselves.

7. There are many reasons why parents don't follow through. Some are mentioned here so that you will be aware of them.

CHAPTER SIX

❧

GET MOVING!

A BOOK SUCH AS THIS WOULDN'T BE complete without a chapter about exercising. As you already know, physical education classes in schools are progressively getting shorter and shorter, with some schools even cutting the subject out altogether. This being so, it's important that in addition to encouraging healthy eating habits in your child, you should also try to incorporate regular exercise into your family's activities.

At this point, you may feel a bit overwhelmed by all of the ideas and suggestions presented here. Perhaps you are even considering skipping this chapter because it seems like too much for you to deal with. This is certainly understandable. You've been hit with a lot of information all at once. In addition, you've been asked to question just about every idea about food that you grew up with, in most cases going against the current social practices. Now you're being asked to think about exercise. Perhaps you're even wondering if I'm a little crazy for bringing up yet another activity to add to your already full list of new things to try.

If you're feeling like this, it's okay. You are not a bad person for not wanting to continue reading even though you know this will benefit your child. You are simply a busy person who is being asked to make a lot of changes that are unfamiliar to most people. That said, I would encourage you to continue reading this chapter. While reading, constantly remind yourself that you don't have to use even one suggestion presented in this chapter. You are simply reading to become informed. There is no pressure to implement anything described here.

Look at this as an exploration of activities that you may or may not decide to use in the future. Do not put any pressure on yourself to follow through here. You already have enough to do with helping your child to eat healthy. And though you may find it difficult to believe, when it's the right time, the exercise portion of your child's life will take care of itself. Your part in this is to simply become aware that the activities outlined in this chapter exist. And when your child is ready, you can pull this book out again and begin offering helpful suggestions. For now, just read on and remind yourself that you are not planning to use any of these tips immediately.

To begin, one of the most important things you can do for your child is to introduce a regular exercise program. If you start early in your child's life, exercise will become a way of life, rather than a desperate chore to be undertaken *after* weight gain. In the same way that healthy eating will eventually become part of your child's life, exercising will as well.

There are two types of exercise on which you should try to concentrate. The first is a regular three-time-a-week formal program that involves consciously planning time to exercise, while the other is more informal and impromptu. Though providing your child with a formal exercise program may seem rigid, you are in fact introducing your child to a habit that will grow with him or her into adulthood. In the same way that your child may have a habit of watching television or sitting in front of the computer, exercise can eventually become one of those activities your child engages in without conscious thought.

As with healthy eating, to introduce your child to a regular exercise program, you will need to be involved in initiating the activity. This can be accomplished in several ways depending on the age of your child. If your child is a preteen, he or she may simply ask to come along when you announce that you've decided to start walking or jogging regularly. If this is so, do not push your child when you are walking or running. You may need to move slower than you'd like and that's okay. This exercising period is about your child, not you. You can always go to the gym later or exercise in another way when your child is not around. Simply encourage your child without demanding or pushing that he or she move faster.

Similarly, if your child tires out after only a few minutes, let him or her know that it's okay. At this point, any exercise is better than none at all. You may want to set manageable goals for your next outing but do so without pressure. Say something like "Maybe next time we can try to make it to that funny-looking tree over there." Notice that there is no pressure here, as the tree (or other object) is only a few extra feet from where you ended. Do not try to get your child to walk an extra mile. This will only cause frustration that will result in your child quitting the exercise program out of fear of disappointing you.

Also, though you may be tempted to measure how long you and your child exercise, avoid doing this in the beginning. The more casual you can keep your exercise periods, the less likely your child is to abandon them. On the other hand, your exercise periods should be consistent. Choose three days a week when you know your child can join you and begin exercising. Let your child know that this is your exercise time and that he or she is welcome to join you. Even if your child decides not to participate, go anyway. Your consistency will be a lesson for your child whether or not he or she joins you.

In the same way that it took a little while for your child to get accustomed to your new eating routine, it may take several weeks before your child decides to join you. You will need to be patient and understanding. Do not pressure your child for any reason. Saying things like "You should get out there and exercise, too," will only cause your child to view exercising as a chore. Similarly, if you constantly complain before your exercise period, your child will share your dread of physical activity. Do not complain. Simply suck it up. Go out and walk. If your child asks you if you're tired, you can explain that even though you are tired, you like the benefits you are getting from exercising so that makes it worthwhile.

Feel free to discuss those benefits and the progress you have made while exercising. For example, if you have more energy and stamina, share this with your child. But, again, avoid dictating to your child what he or she should do. Simply stick to discussing the benefits YOU are experiencing. Do not overwhelm your child with every good point about exercising. Choose one or two benefits and share them on your exercise days in a casual manner. Then, let it drop. If your child has questions, feel free to answer them. If not, continue exercising as you have been. Eventually, your activities will serve as a powerful example for you child to imitate. Again, you need to be consistent with your exercising. This will teach your child that regular exercise is vital to good health and seeing you do it will encourage your child to join in.

The second type of exercise that you can incorporate into your child's life involves changing your family routines to include physical activity. If, for instance, it is your family's custom to see a movie on Saturday afternoon, why not take a hike, go bowling, play miniature golf, or even a good old-fashioned game of touch football? If these suggestions aren't quite right for your family, then find something that is. Does your family enjoy swimming? Ice hockey? Baseball? Basketball? Playing at the playground? Walking in the park? Water skiing? Scuba diving? Playing tennis? Whatever it is, initiate a family activity at least twice a month. Not only will your child come to enjoy exercising but your family will learn to play together in a healthy way.

While all of the previously mentioned pastimes can obviously be considered exercise, there are others that you may not have considered when thinking of physical activities. For instance, walking around an amusement park or a large mall will provide your child with physical activity in a potentially enjoyable way. Be sure, of course, to avoid eating areas and food courts. Another way for you to give your child exercise is to begin parking your car farther away from the entrance to wherever it is you are going. Again, this may seem to be a small amount of exercise but it's still more than your child was getting before.

Why try so hard to incorporate physical activity into your child's day? Think about this. According to a 2010 report at the Center for Disease Control and Prevention, only 20.4 percent of the U.S. population met the Physical Activity Guidelines for both aerobic and muscle-strengthening physical activity. Furthermore, as stated in the organization's 2010 National Health Survey, "according to the 2008 federal physical activity guidelines for aerobic activity, 33 percent of adults were inactive, 20 percent of adults were insufficiently active, and 47 percent were sufficiently active based on their participation in leisure-time physical activity." Now, contrast this with the fact that in most American households, television is on for seven and a half hours per day. *That is not a typo:* per day.

Now, consider this: 33 percent of adults are completely sedentary during their free time while 20 percent rarely exercise. With television and computers being such predominant parts of American life, it's not difficult to imagine what these adults do in their spare time. The alarming part about these statistics is the fact that exercise or physical activity is not a part of life for almost half of all adults. In the same way that eating has taken over American life, exercise is slowly being thrown out, contributing to a very dangerous health environment.

Once again, by trying to incorporate exercise into your child's life, you are swimming against the tide of the habits practiced by most Americans. As Marie Winn points out in *The Plug-In Drug*, there are families whose philosophy is "no-television-ever." One mother Winn profiles discusses the opposition she faces as a no-television-ever mom. "We have been accused many times of culturally depriving our children by not having a TV. You'd be amazed at how emotional and angry people can become when you express the idea that you don't approve of television. It's worse than attacking motherhood or apple pie. We take our four children to concerts and museums and don't feel they're deprived of culture. On the contrary, I'm well pleased with their physical, mental, and emotional development—they're active, eager, curious, independent doers. They love to read, do well in school, and have good imaginations. They never run out of things to do."

Another parent expands on this. "Once in a while we'll rent a set for a special occasion like a big sports event. But for us, television is like junk food—a once-in-a-while thing."

Chances are pretty good that you will face the same sort of opposition when trying to change your child's eating habits and encouraging physical activity. Though both of these are healthy pursuits and you may not expect that others would be critical of such an undertaking, there is a good chance that you will experience resistance.

What does this mean for you and your child? Quite simply, if the US government faces great difficulty when trying to change American habits—as it has when attempting to get Americans to use seatbelts while driving, or to quit smoking—it is naïve to think that you won't, too. However, both of the abovementioned behaviors have been changed. Seat-belt and no-smoking laws are now common, and are met with widespread public approval. Inroads have also been made against drunk driving and driving while texting. It can be done.

Remember that when making an attempt to change your own lifestyle, you influence others to think about their own eating and exercise habits. Many people are uncomfortable with this and may unconsciously try to sabotage your efforts.

Americans are innovative, "get 'er done," people, in love with efficiency. This has both positive and negative aspects. We sometimes try to apply the principles of ease and efficiency to areas of our life that call for other virtues; namely, patience and discipline. Weight-loss is one such area. Instead of changing exercise and diet behaviors, which takes time and effort, most Americans are easily convinced that the "easy, efficient" thing to do is to pop a pill.

The diet-pill industry takes advantage of this tendency. Whatever diet pill happens to be the flavor of the month is all but guaranteed to make millions, if not billions of dollars, for its manufacturer. Despite possible side effects and even fatalities associated with the use of drugs, millions of Americans continue to look toward pills—not dietary changes and exercise—to lose weight.

While this may seem to be simply a part of American life, let's think about the message being sent to children when adults use pills to lose weight. By using diet pills, an individual is buying into and implicitly supporting a false notion and one that is the dream of everyone who wishes to lose weight—that we could each simply take a pill and maintain a healthy weight without watching what we eat or exercising. That's every dieter's dream—the "magic pill" that will allow this. Yet, diet pill manufacturers are careful to promote their products as a means of *supplementing* weight loss efforts and caution that the pills should be used in conjunction with a healthy eating plan. In other words, whether or not you take the pills, you are still supposed to eat healthily. This is a far cry from the ideas that most Americans have about diet pills.

To put it bluntly, many Americans are in denial about what it takes to manage one's weight loss and exercise efforts. The use of diet pills is evidence of this. Rather than simply eating well and exercising, many people choose to swallow pills that may have dangerous side effects. In the nineties, the drugs Fen/Phen and Redux were introduced. Designed to enhance brain chemical activity, the diet drugs gained widespread attention almost immediately. According to one medical expert, the diet pills provided a 10 to 20 percent boost to weight loss efforts. But some patients actually gained weight on the medication because they felt they could eat as much as they wanted— the pill would do the rest. As Dr. Ken Goodrick of Baylor College of Medicine pointed out in a personal communication, "A medication can help a person resist the temptation to overeat, but it can't prevent all emotional overeating, unless the pill is held carefully between the teeth. In most treatment programs, there always a few who fail to control eating, and who gain weight." Clearly, some "dieters" on Fen/Phen believed that taking the drug without making necessary lifestyle changes was all they needed to do—how very disappointed they must have been.

If disappointment was all that those who took the Fen/Phen and Redux diet pills suffered, it wouldn't have been so bad. However, users dramatically increased their chances of contracting primary pulmonary hypertension (elevated blood pressure affecting the pulmonary artery) by as much as 30 percent. Primary pulmonary hypertension is a sometimes-fatal disease that damages the heart when not enough oxygen is pumped to it. If this happened and you were lucky enough to find it in time, you would have a choice—an oxygen pump to help you breathe or a dangerous lung transplant. That is, of course, if you were lucky enough to have survived. An article in *The New England Journal of Medicine* reported that a twenty-nine-year-old woman who took Fen/Phen for twenty-three days died of pulmonary hypertension. Additional side effects included brain damage, severe diarrhea, extreme mood swings, shortness of breath, racing heart, irritability, depression, impotence, diminished libido, headaches, dry mouth, drowsiness, insomnia, fatigue, vivid dreams, hallucinations, anxiety, and manic-depressive reactions.

Despite this, in 1996, Fen/Phen was the second fastest growing drug, making $191 million that year for its manufacturer. Over a three-year period, prescriptions for the drug rose from 60,000 to about 1.1 million. And, in the first five months of its introduction, doctors wrote 1.2 million prescriptions for Redux, with sales totaling more than $20 million a month. Wyeth-Ayerst, the makers of Redux, estimated that more than two million people took the drug during its fifteen months of existence. Couple that with the four million who have used Pondimin—the brand name for fenfluramine—since 1973, with most being in recent years, and you have an idea of exactly how unwilling to embrace new eating habits Americans can be in their weight-loss and exercise efforts.

On September 15, 1997, the FDA issued a statement urging individuals to stop taking the drugs after evaluating the results of nearly

300 patients' heart tests. The results showed that 92 of the 291 people studied had damaged heart valves even though they had no symptoms. Following that, the FDA requested that drug manufacturers voluntarily recall their products. Both companies agreed.

Even though these drugs have been recalled, there are others out there. Unfortunately, it's human nature to seek out seemingly easier solutions to problems. Americans are constantly on the look out for "softer" ways to lose weight that don't involve a lot of effort. Add to this the fact that drug manufacturers work overtime to make these diet pills attractive to consumers and you have an idea of just how popular these dangerous diet pills can be.

There is no doubt that you will need to be firm and strong in your decisions. No matter how much anyone urges you to forego your healthy new way of life, you will need to forge ahead with your plans, simply remembering that you are bucking the trend in order to better your child's life. You will learn more about how to deal with this societal resistance in Chapter Eight, but for now consider that the heaviest youngsters are more than twice as likely as the thinnest to die prematurely, before age fifty-five, of illness or a self-inflicted injury. Youngsters with a condition called pre-diabetes are at almost double the risk of dying before fifty-five, and those with high blood pressure are at some increased risk. But obesity is the factor most closely associated with an early death, according to medical research.

Helping your child to take responsibility for his or her eating habits is one of the most important lessons you can teach, but it's one that too many adults in our society haven't learned. A litigious New York maintenance worker who, at 5 feet 10 inches, found that he weighed 270 pounds claimed in court that he and a number of other obese and ill New Yorkers who eat fast food four or five times a week had no idea that so much greasy, salty food was bad for them. Even after suffering a heart attack, the plaintiff kept eating the unhealthy food sold by these fast-food restaurants, claiming the restaurant chains did not properly disclose the ingredients of their food and the risks of eating too much of it.

The idea that Americans can sue fast-food companies for choices and decisions they, themselves, are making seems outlandish and has even been ridiculed by late-night comedians, but lawsuits like this are becoming common. However, blaming someone else does not help anyone to take responsibility for his or her own choices. Without responsibility there is no room for change. So, while it may be tempting to blame fast-food restaurants because the food tastes so good, or even your mother for baking those cookies your child can't resist, blaming others will not help to improve your child's eating habits.

Legislation was passed recently to force fast-food restaurants to list the ingredients and calories in their establishments. Though the intention of this law was to discourage overeating, it does not appear to have helped. More Americans than ever are overweight, and fast-food chains are making even greater profits. In the third quarter of 2011, McDonald's profits rose 9 percent. It was the ninth consecutive quarter that profits rose, making the company's net income $1.5 billion. Similarly, midway through 2012, Burger King's profits were up by 60 percent, contributing to a net income of $48.2 million.

Considered strictly from a healthy-eating point of view, these figures are upsetting (although to the shareholders of these companies they represent good news). However, it's important to realize that each person who walks through the doors of a fast-food restaurant has a choice about what he or she will eat. And while many of these restaurants are adding items lower in fat and calories to their menus, the majority of people who eat there are not taking advantage of them or are mixing them with high-calorie foods. Adding croutons, high-fat dressing, and cheese to a salad, for example, is nearly as unhealthy as eating french fries, yet most people feel better about the salad.

Although numerous obesity-prevention programs do exist, they function in a piecemeal fashion instead of in the holistic, consistent manner that is necessary for success. A December 20, 2011 study published at the Department of Health & Human Services Agency for Healthcare Research and Quality website analyzed twenty childhood obesity prevention programs. Most of the programs were school-based and "did not include interventions conducted in other settings, such as home, community, built-environment, and primary care," according to the researchers. The researchers note that "A growing consensus in the field is that comprehensive intervention programs, those that involve multiple sectors in our society or that target multiple factors affecting energy balance behaviors, are needed to fight the obesity epidemic in the US." Your involvement at the parental level, then, may be one of the "multiple sectors" that are the vital, but too often missing, components that can make the difference in your child's health.

Things to Remember

1. Exercise is important to help your child stay healthy.

2. In the beginning, try to keep it casual. Never bribe, shame, or otherwise coerce your child to exercise.

3. Set a good example. Begin exercising when and where your child can observe you.

4. Most children don't get enough exercise at school and some don't even have any at all, so it's important for you to make this a priority in both of your lives.

5. Chances are that you will face some sort of opposition if only because other parents do not want to make the effort. Keep doing it anyway!

6. Overweight youngsters are more than twice as likely to die younger.

7. Be consistent.

CHAPTER SEVEN

⛬

EXTREMES

WHILE MANY OF THE TIPS PRESENTED THROUGHOUT this book will help overweight children with unhealthy eating habits, there are exceptions to this. Children and teens with eating disorders require special assistance from professionals. This chapter will help you to decide whether or not your child has an eating disorder. It is not, however, designed as a substitute for professional help.

It is also important to realize that even if your child doesn't exhibit any of the symptoms or behaviors outlined in this chapter, he or she is not immune from developing one in the future. Therefore, careful attention to the material presented here is vital to your child's continued good health.

Anorexia Nervosa is known as the "starving sickness." Those afflicted with this disease have an intense fear of eating, often resulting in starvation. Characteristically, anorexics are extremely underweight, often concerned about achieving perfection in all areas of their lives, and intensely afraid of weight gain. Oftentimes these individuals are obsessed with food—even looking through recipes and cooking food for others—yet rarely ever eating. Socially, anorexics are withdrawn, irritable, even depressed. In most cases those suffering from *anorexia nervosa* have distorted body images, unable to see exactly how thin and emaciated their bodies have become.

Bulimia Nervosa is an eating disorder characterized by eating large amounts and then getting rid of the food either through exercise, use of diuretics and/or laxatives, and/or vomiting. In general, people who suffer from bulimia maintain an average weight through these "purging" methods. Similarly to anorexics, bulimics may withdraw from society, may be irritable and depressed, and are secretive about eating patterns.

Nonpurging Bulimia is an eating disorder characterized by episodes of eating large amounts of food but without the activity of purging.

Food addiction is defined as a physical and emotional addiction to certain food substances—usually sugar, flour, fats, and sometimes wheat—that results in overwhelming cravings for foods containing these substances. In addition to a physical dependence, food addicts also experience an emotional dependence, which causes them to become extremely attached to food. Other characteristics include social withdrawal, irritability, and depression.

Though some symptoms of these three types of eating disorders differ, there are certain characteristics that are similar to all of them. Following is a discussion about the warning signs for eating disorders in general. Included will be a quiz for you to take to determine whether or not your child is suffering from an eating disorder.

One of the biggest signs of an eating disorder is secretive eating. While it may be common for children to eat foods without their parents' knowledge during the school day or on social occasions outside the home, this is not "secretive" eating, per se. A child ashamed of over- or under-eating often chooses to eat in private. This is especially the case for a child suffering from bulimia. Directly after a meal, the child will head right to the bathroom or exercise area to rid his or her body of the food eaten. A child or teen with an eating disorder may attempt to sneak food into the house and hide it to eat in secret later. Since a significant element of eating disorders involves shame while eating, it is easy to understand how secretive eating plays a part.

To avoid encouraging your child to eat in private, try to serve structured meals at the kitchen or dining room table. Do not encourage your child to bring food to his or her room. On the other hand, it is not a good idea to go in the opposite direction either. If you try to forbid your child from eating certain foods, your child will feel the need to sneak these foods into the house. Remember, your plan is to only bring healthy food into the house. Do not make strict rules regarding these foods, unless, of course, you are advised to by a doctor or counselor who is aware of your specific situation.

If you find that your child is sneaking food, it is even more important that you de-emotionalize food. By admonishing your child for sneaking food, you will cause him or her to associate excitement, rebellion, and/or freedom with eating. This will not only associate emotions with eating but it will also cause your child to look to food for these feelings. Also, just because your child eats in secret, does not automatically mean he or she suffers from an eating disorder. Rather, you will need to monitor your child's activities and the frequency or extent of them to make that determination.

For example, if your child sneaks food only occasionally, then this can be considered to be normal childhood behavior; but if you find this to be a weekly or even a biweekly event, then there may be cause for concern. How do you know if your child is sneaking food? It's really quite simple. Keep your eyes and ears open. Are there food wrappers in his or her room? Can you hear crinkling sounds from bags? Does he or she leave the bedroom with food stains on skin or clothes? While it is not a good idea to violate your child's privacy, there is no harm in paying attention to his or her actions.

The decision about whether or not to confront your child is a very personal one and should not be made without careful thought. While it is important for your child to be honest about his or her eating habits, you cannot force a conversation such as this. Rather than yelling at your child, it will be necessary to create a calm and accepting atmosphere for your child to feel safe. If secretive eating seems to be a large part of your child's life or if you feel uncomfortable bringing up the subject, you may want to consider seeking help from a family counselor or psychiatrist. With the help of a professional you will have a safe, neutral environment in which to discuss your concerns with your child.

Another eating disorder indicator is a high level of emotional dependence on food. You've already read about the many roles that food plays in society and you've written about your child's behavior. Now, you will need to determine if your child is simply exhibiting normal societal behavior or if there is a deeper problem. The most effective way to do this is to see the level of dependence your child has around food. When your child is upset, for example, does he or she turn right to food? What is the first thing he or she does when getting up on a weekend day? What about before going to sleep? In what way does your child celebrate? If you answered food and/or eating to any of these questions, then you will need to examine the frequency of your child's reactions.

For instance, how many times during the week does your child seem to be upset? Is he or she moody and/or depressed? Does he or she regularly spend hours at a time in his or her room alone? Is your child very often alone? How regularly does your child spend time outside of school with friends? If you had to use one word to describe your child's emotional state, what would that word be? In general, depression is a symptom of eating disorders. Though a biological illness all its own, depression often occurs with eating disorders. It may take a professional to determine whether or not your child is suffering from an eating disorder or from depression.

Another sign that your child may be suffering from an eating disorder is a strong preoccupation with body image and size. While a certain amount of concern about body size is a normal part of adolescence, too much emphasis may indicate the presence of an eating disorder. Think about how many times your child looks in the mirror throughout the day. Does it seem excessive? Children who never look in the mirror are a cause for concern, too. Either extreme is unhealthy.

Pay attention to the subtle messages your child sends out about his or her body. For example, is he or she constantly saying negative things about his or her size? Are there certain body parts that your child continually focuses on in a negative way? Following are a few examples that, when repeated, may be cause for concern:

- "My hips are so big and ugly. I could never wear that."
- "I'm too fat to be a cheerleader."
- "My muscles aren't big enough to go out for the football team."
- "My legs are too heavy and disgusting."
- "My stomach is too fat."
- "I hate my body."
- "I'm so ugly and disgusting. I can't stand myself."

Though your child may use different words, notice what he or she is saying. If you have the opportunity to see your child interact with friends, you can listen for clues then, too. Listen to what they say about their bodies. Some of these messages may be disguised as discussions related to clothes and/or sports. Does your child constantly talk about clothes that he or she can't wear due to various body issues? When shopping for school clothes, does your child make negative comments about his or her appearance? If so, you may want to think about all of these types of comments your child makes. A negative comment occasionally about his or her body size is nothing to be concerned about but when it happens consistently, it may indicate a problem.

Similarly, another warning sign may come in the form of your child's friends. Do any of them have eating disorders? Is one very thin or very overweight? In general, people with eating disorders tend to seek out others in the same situation. In the same way that children choose friends based on common interests, those with disordered eating habits are generally attracted to each other. Though you may have become accustomed to seeing your child's friends, take a second look at them and their habits. Do their actions match any of those described in this book? If so, this may indicate your child has or is on the way to developing an eating disorder.

As with much of the information discussed here, it is important not to forbid your child from seeing his or her friend(s) if you suspect the presence of an eating disorder. Remember, that will only make this friend more attractive. For right now, simply follow the suggestions in this book until you can seek the advice of a professional. A professional will help you to determine how to approach your child about this issue. Since each child is different, it will be necessary to find a professional to help with this situation.

Another indicator that your child may have an eating disorder is erratic behavior. If your once calm and easygoing child has turned moody, irritable, and withdrawn, he or she may be suffering from an eating disorder. Some of these symptoms may be normal preteen behavior, however; therefore, it will be necessary to observe your child's actions over several days or even weeks before making a final determination.

In line with this, you may also want to be aware of your child's overall personality traits. For example, was your child once flexible in his or her routine but now seems to be rigid and unbending in daily routines and activities? Or, does your once-easygoing child seem to be regularly in pursuit of perfectionism both at school and at home? Does your child seem to spend hours on his or her homework, not quitting until it's perfect? Though most parents would love to see their children overly enthusiastic about their homework, taken to the extreme of perfectionism, this may be the telltale sign of an eating disorder and needs to be considered along with the other symptoms discussed here as an overall pattern of behavior.

The development of rituals around eating behaviors is another symptom of an eating disorder. If this is the case, you may notice that your child will need to have things in a certain order or form at each meal or every time he or she eats. Your child will most likely never vary from the established forms. Examples of this type of behavior include: eating three popcorn kernels at a time, never eating "beige" foods, only eating items in pairs, never eating more than three different types of food, only eating while listening to the same song at every meal, watching a certain television show while eating a specific food, only reading or doing homework if a particular food is present, never eating with certain people or being unwilling to eat without a particular toy or object.

Additional symptoms may include a preoccupation with shopping for food as well as shopping in general, a strong need to present a pulled-together appearance, difficulty making decisions, unusual self-consciousness about body size, and a fascination with exercise.

Though every attempt has been made to include the most common eating disorder symptoms, it is impossible to include a complete list, as each child is different and may exhibit only one of those mentioned. In general, however, if you notice that your child demonstrates at least two or three of the behaviors outlined in this chapter, he or she may have or be at high risk for an eating disorder. If this is the case, you should seek professional help immediately as eating disorders do not heal themselves. It will require work on both your part and that of your child.

Following is a quiz that may assist you in determining whether or not your child has an eating disorder:

- Does he or she seem to talk about food most of the time?
- Does it sometimes seem as if he or she feels driven to eat?
- Has he or she ever lied about how much he or she has eaten?
- As time has goes on, has his or her eating (whether that means eating either more or less) become more pronounced?
- Does he or she either frequently step on the scale or completely avoid it?
- Does it seem as if he or she feels out of control when eating? Does he or she seemingly try to eat as much as possible in a short amount of time?
- Has his or her body size ever affected participation in certain activities?
- When he or she has not eaten a favorite food in a while, does he or she seem to be angry or depressed?
- Has he or she ever eaten before going out for a meal so as not to eat a lot in front of others?

- Does it seem as if food is the only thing that never lets your child down?

Take a few days or even weeks to determine the answers to these questions. Keep track of the answers. If you notice that you can answer "yes" to at least four of these, then it's most likely that your child is suffering from an eating disorder. Also, think carefully before answering each question. For example, when determining how much your child seems to talk about food, you need to be aware that in certain instances it is normal behavior for a child to have thoughts of food. As you know, birthdays are associated with eating cake and holidays with baking cookies. If your child only thinks about food during these times, this is likely a societal reaction or one based on personal history, rather than anything that indicates the presence of an eating disorder.

On the other hand, if your child seems to talk about food when there seems to be no apparent reason, then he or she may be showing signs of an eating disorder. Similarly, if your child seems to turn to food when something goes wrong, then he or she may be exhibiting concrete signs of an eating disorder.

Perhaps one of the most difficult things you will be asked to do in this chapter is to evaluate the answers you have given to this quiz. To do so, it will be necessary for you to try and view your child in an objective manner. As a parent, it is your natural instinct to want to protect your child. Because of this, you may be tempted to minimize the answers or try to present your child in a more positive light than is realistic. Try to avoid this as it is necessary for your answers to be accurate in order to make a fair determination of your child's eating habits. To do this, you may want to enlist the help of a trusted relative or friend.

When deciding on someone to help you, the most important thing is to choose someone whose opinion you trust. Remember, if you are asking for an opinion, you may hear something that you do not like. This being so, you will need to find someone whom you trust enough to give you an honest answer. For example, if you have always hated the way your best friend criticizes everything, then he or she may not be the right choice as your shared history will prevent you from listening objectively to her opinions. Finding someone who is neutral and whom you trust to tell the truth is the best way to go.

CHAPTER EIGHT

❧

LOOKING TOWARD THE FUTURE

IT IS SAFE TO SAY THAT YOU'VE "digested" some very difficult truths about both society's emotional eating habits and also those of your own family. Hopefully, you've even completed several of the exercises outlined in this book and are beginning to experience some significant changes in the way you relate to your child where food is concerned. If this is the case, take a moment to congratulate yourself. What you have accomplished is no small miracle by any means. Quite the opposite, you have done one of the most difficult tasks anyone can—making a major lifestyle change.

If you haven't yet gotten around to doing the exercises outlined in these pages, please take some time to do so as the results will more than be worth the effort. Though it may seem overwhelming or scary to take that first step, realize that you only have to make one small change in order to begin. Why not take ten minutes right now to take action? Remember, if you devoted ten minutes each day to helping your child take the emotion out of food, you would see dramatic results in no time. If you can't seem to find ten minutes out of your day, then you need to consider what activities you are participating in that are more important than the health of your child. You get to choose where you devote your energies. It's vital that you consider this idea when determining whether or not you can spare the time.

If you have already begun making changes, you've probably faced some resistance both within your family and in your community. Though it may not be easy, it is necessary for you to continue in the direction you are moving toward. Again, remind yourself that you are fighting for your child's life and future. Isn't a little discomfort worth that?

In your childhood you probably weren't given specific tools to deal with social discomfort or taught how to set specific boundaries without alienating people. Unfortunately, when faced with uncomfortable situations, most people choose one of two options—running away or getting belligerent. Neither is very effective in developing or maintaining healthy relationships.

Those who react by running away have made it more difficult for themselves to face these people in the future; while those who become belligerent push others away, thus also making it challenging to maintain relationships. If you have already reacted either way, realize that you did the best you could at the time but be sure to continue reading so that you will have additional options available to you.

Let's take an example wherein your child is invited to go to the movies with a family that regularly buys several bags of candy for each child in the group. Having made serious progress in changing your child's eating habits, you are reluctant to allow your child to go with this family. Though your first instinct may be to create an excuse, this may not be the most effective way of handling the situation. If done on a regular basis, you will alienate this family; and, besides, a made-up excuse is dishonest and cowardly. Another option is to discuss the family's eating habits directly with the parents. Though this, too, may seem logical, it may not have the effect you desire. While it may be possible in a perfect world to discuss the family's eating habits without making them defensive, chances are good that they will be offended by what they'll rightly consider to be your criticism of their eating habits.

Rather than the two examples discussed, consider a third option that involves directly talking to one of the parents about your concerns for your child's health. Use only the word "I" never "you," and explain how dangerous these foods have become to your child's current and future health. If you feel comfortable enough, you may discuss some of the changes you have already made. Even though this course of action may seem similar to the previous one mentioned, it is not. In the previous approach, you are commenting directly about the family's eating habits whereas in this one you are simply talking about your concerns for your child and the steps you are taking to help him or her.

The previous example invites defensiveness on the part of the family while the third option enlists assistance by honestly sharing *your* experience. It is a rare parent who would go against the wishes another parent has for his or her child. If by some chance you do find that this family has ignored your expressed wishes, you may want to reconsider whether or not to accept any more movie invitations for your child that come from them. Play dates that take place on your home "turf," where your rules and boundaries can be enforced, may be a better choice in future.

If you are reading this book, you know that your child has a problem, and you want to help find a solution. If you have read this far, you know that part of that solution involves lifestyle changes.

You have so far committed to change some of the activities you spend your time on—and the people you choose to spend time with may also have to change. One reason for this may be that your former associates may not share your commitment to a healthy lifestyle. They may even offer resistance to it, whether because they don't understand it or even because they flat-out disagree with it. Either way, your child's health is at stake. A more positive reason that your companions may change is due to the fact that you are participating in different activities; and, therefore, you will be meeting new people who share your new lifestyle. Neither group of companions is right or wrong, good or bad. This change is simply a result of the growth you are experiencing.

Similarly, if you have already begun making some of the changes described here, you are probably creating new and healthy rituals for your family that may be unfamiliar to those around you. For example, if you've chosen to have an active birthday party, such as organizing a craft or sporting event for the children, rather than a passive one, such as going to a fast-food restaurant or seeing a movie, then not only are you helping your child to develop healthier habits but you are assisting other children to do the same as well. Though other parents may find it strange that you've decided to take your child and his or her friends horseback riding or to an indoor play center rather than the usual trip to the local fast-food establishment, make no mistake that they will learn a new way of celebrating birthdays from your efforts.

Remember: it isn't necessary to develop an all-or-nothing attitude where your child's activities are concerned. For instance, if your child is over the age of three, he or she has become accustomed to celebrating his or her birthday with cake. To suddenly discontinue this activity may create confusion, even resentment about your family's new way of life. Rather than discontinue the cake immediately, consider a compromise. With today's innovations in food creation, most children will not even notice a lower-in-fat substitute for the cake. Or, if you're feeling especially adventurous, you may even consider a lower-calorie option with frosting that is drizzled on lightly, rather than spread completely over the cake. Whatever you decide, be sure to consider your child's wishes as the point is not to spoil the festivities but simply to begin to develop healthy ways of celebrating that don't always involve food.

Even if you are the most committed person in the world, at some point you will feel a decrease in your enthusiasm. This is only natural. To help you prepare for this, following are eight suggestions to keep you motivated. Once again, choose the ones that work for you and your family.

Eight Tips to Keep You Motivated

1. **Read something daily that supports your new way of life.**
    Every one of us has a built-in "forgetter." This means that if you do not constantly reinforce new ideas, you will inevitably forget why it's important to continue to progress in the new direction. To help with this, find something to read each day, even if it's a sentence or two from this book. Not only will you see this information differently but you will also remind yourself about the importance of continuing in a healthy direction.

2. **Seek out others who are living the sort of life you are working toward.**
    One of the best ways to reinforce your new lifestyle habits is to surround yourself with others who are in agreement with what you are trying to do. While it isn't necessary to find someone who perfectly mirrors what you do, seeking out others with similar views will keep you going when your

energy begins to wane. In the same way that it is easier to keep a commitment to work out regularly if you have a partner, seeking others with similar lifestyles will provide you with the same type of motivation. Support groups can be found in many community guides or local newspapers.

3. **Constantly remind yourself that you are helping your child.**

As with anything in life, there will come a time when making changes in your lifestyle will seem overwhelming and difficult. It is for this reason that you will need to remind yourself on a daily, if not hourly or minute-by-minute, basis that all of your effort is worth it because you are helping to change your child's life for the better. Even more, realize that by establishing permanent changes in your child's life, you are influencing future generations as well. In other words, you are not only changing your child's eating habits but you may also be influencing those of your future grandchildren and even great-grandchildren. Certainly, the effort you are putting into this is worth all of that.

4. **Keep a journal of your progress.**

Throughout this book, writing has been encouraged as a means of developing deeper understanding. By continuing the patterns you've already established, you can create a concrete reminder of the progress you've made. Even if writing daily in a journal is out of the question, consider taking a weekly inventory on Saturday or Sunday when your schedule may not be as hectic. Simply writing a sentence or two about the changes you've seen in your child's eating habits will help you to remember exactly how far you've come. Remember, humans have a built in "forgetter" that makes it difficult to keep your accomplishments in mind. You can counteract this by writing about your progress.

5. Get in the habit of planning ahead.

You've already read that planning meals ahead will prevent spur-of-the-moment emotional overeating. Now, it's time to put this concept into action. The first few times that you attempt to prepare a meal in advance or pack a lunch the night before, you may feel overwhelmed; but it's important to realize that each time you do this it will get easier. Generally, it takes 21 days to develop a habit, with each attempt contributing to making a permanent lifestyle change. This being so, it is important to get over the initial adjustment "hump." Hang in there and it will get easier.

6. Create a scrapbook of inspirational sayings and photos.

Similar to a journal charting your progress, a scrapbook of sayings and photos that you find inspirational will provide you with a valuable resource when you feel discouraged. Though you may want to purchase a special book for this, you can simply paste or tape things into a notebook if that's what works for you. It doesn't matter what it looks like as long as you can easily access the information it contains. You may even find that you enjoy searching out inspirational quotes and photos. So, go ahead and rip up magazines, books, and newspapers. Print out things from the Internet or take the lyrics from your favorite song. Whatever it is that inspires you, add it to your scrapbook.

7. **Regularly reward yourself for a job well done**.

Making a major lifestyle change takes an incredible amount of effort. It is hard work; and as with any difficult task, you need to reward yourself for your commitment. Treat yourself to a massage. Buy a new pair of shoes or that sweater that you've had your eye on. Go to that concert or show that you've always wanted to. Take a long drive in the country or buy a special book or magazine. Whatever it is that's important to you, treat yourself! Be careful, however, not to involve food in this celebration in any way. This will counteract the hard work you've done.

8. **Reward your child for a job well done**.

In the same way that you need a reward, your child does as well. Though you need to stay away from food-related activities, you may want to take your child on a special outing. Spend time doing something your child enjoys or introduce him or her to a new activity—build or make something with him or her, or let him or her teach you something. Be careful, however, not to do this on a daily or weekly basis, as this will once again tie emotions with food-related behavior. Save the rewards for unexpected times that don't relate to any food-related accomplishment. Rather, view the rewards as a means of supporting your child in his or her new lifestyle—NOT as a means of rewarding food-related behavior.

Now that you have some concrete suggestions about how to keep motivated in your new lifestyle, it's time for you to create two of your own. Taking some of the suggestions previously mentioned, write two ways of your own that will keep you going when the task seems difficult. As you write, be sure to consider your family and current lifestyle. For example, don't create something so unrealistic that you won't be able to follow through. If, for instance, finances are tight, don't suggest taking a major vacation as the impracticality of the event will automatically make it impossible for you to use. So, go ahead, write two of your own. Then, try them.

As you continue with your new lifestyle changes, it's important to always keep the end result of your efforts in mind. By making healthy changes in your child's life, you are enhancing his or her life as well as vastly improving the quality of life. As a formerly overweight child, I can point to hundreds of things that I missed out on. I can never recapture these experiences and will always live with the pain of missing out on so many things that normal weight children take for granted. As a parent reading this book, you have an opportunity to change your child's whole life. Rather than live a life based in unhappiness, your child can be a happy, productive, energetic, and enthusiastic member of society. The suggestions in this book and your commitment will help you to make this a reality.

RECOMMENDED READING

Food Politics: How the Food Industry Influences Nutrition and Health
by Marion Nestle
Second Edition, Revised Edition
(University of California Press, 2007)

*Food Fight: The Inside Story of the Food Industry, America's Obesity
Crisis, and What We Can Do About It*
by Kelly D. Brownell and Katherine Battle Horgen
(McGraw-Hill, 2004)

Your Child's Weight: Helping without Harming
By Ellyn Satter, MS, RD, LCSW, BCD
(Kelcy Press, 2005)

ONLINE RESOURCES

Online Resources
Help Cure Child Obesity
http://www.helpcurechildobesity.com/

Kids Health
http://kidshealth.org/parent/

My Overweight Child
http://www.myoverweightchild.com/blog/

Official Website of Debbie Danowski, PhD
http://debbiedanowski.com/

RELATED SUPPORT GROUPS

OVEREATERS ANONYMOUS
Overeaters Anonymous World Service Office
PO Box 44020
Rio Rancho, NM 87174-4020
(505) 891-2664
www.oa.org

ANOREXICS AND BULIMICS ANONYMOUS
Anorexics and Bulimics Anonymous
Main PO Box 125
Edmonton, AB T5J 2G9
Canada
(780) 443-6077
2b212steps.org

FAMILIES ANONYMOUS
Families Anonymous
701 Lee St.
Suite 670
Des Plaines, IL 60016
(800) 736-9805
www.familiesanonymous.org

FOOD ADDICTS ANONYMOUS
Food Addicts Anonymous
World Service Office
529 N W Prima Vista Blvd.
#301A
Port St. Lucie, FL 34983
(772) 878-9657
www.foodaddictsanonymous.org

ALSO FROM CENTRAL RECOVERY PRESS

❦

FOR YOUNG ADULTS AND YOUNG READERS

First Star I See
Jaye Andras Caffrey, illustrated by Lynne Adamson
ISBN-13: 978-1-936290-01-7
$12.95 US

The Secret of Willow Ridge: Gabe's Dad Finds Recovery
Helen H. Moore, illustrated by John Blackford
Foreword by Claudia Black, PhD
ISBN-13: 978-0-9818482-0-4
$12.95 US

Mommy's Gone to Treatment

Mommy's Coming Home from Treatment

Denise D. Crosson, PhD, illustrated by Mike Motz
ISBN-13: 978-0-9799869-1-8

ISBN-13: 978-0-9799869-4-9
$14.95 US

Why Is Brian So Fat?

Gary Solomon, PhD Illustrated by Lynne Adamson
ISBN-13: 978-1-936290-74-1

$14.95 US

ABOUT THE AUTHOR

Debbie Danowski, PhD is the author of four popular books about weight loss and food addiction and an associate professor of Media Studies at Sacred Heart University in Fairfield, Connecticut. Her latest book is *The Emotional Eater's Book of Inspiration: 90 Truths You Need to Know to Overcome Your Food Addiction* (Avalon/Marlowe). Her other books include *Why Can't I Stop Eating?* (Hazelden 2000) co-authored with Dr. Pedro Lazaro, *Locked Up for Eating Too Much* (Hazelden 2002), and *The Overeater's Journal* (Hazelden 2004).

Additionally, Dr. Danowski has written more than 100 articles for national and local publications, including *First For Women, Woman's Day* and *Seventeen Magazine,* and served as a contributing writer for *Fairfield County Home* magazine. She has also spoken at countless meetings, seminars, and conferences about weight loss and food addiction, including *Food Addiction 2000*, the first national conference held on the disease.